CORONARY BYPASS SURGERY
Who Needs It?

CORONARY BYPASS SURGERY

Who Needs It?

Siegfried J. Kra, M.D., F.A.C.P.

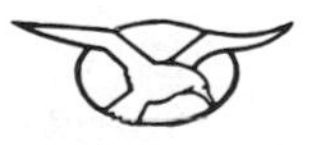

W. W. Norton & Company New York London

Printed in the United States of America.
The text of this book is composed in Janson, with display type set in Zapf International. Composition and manufacturing by The Haddon Craftsmen, Inc.
Book design by Bernard Klein.
First Edition

Library of Congress Cataloging in Publication Data
Kra, Siegfried J.
Coronary bypass surgery.
1. Aortocoronary bypass. 2. Aortocoronary bypass—Decision making. I. Title. [DNLM: 1. Aortocoronary Bypass—popular works. WG 169 K89c]
RD598.K73 1986 617'.412 85-7093

ISBN 0-393-01988-8

W. W. Norton & Company, Inc., 500 Fifth Avenue, New York, N. Y. 10110
W. W. Norton & Company Ltd., 37 Great Russell Street, London WC1B 3NU
1 2 3 4 5 6 7 8 9 0

Dedicated to my patients

Contents

Illustrations

Introduction

EACH year as many as 1.5 million Americans have heart attacks, and there are at least 5 million Americans suffering from angina (coronary artery disease).

Most of these victims ask the pertinent question: "Do I need a stress test, cardiac catheterization, and bypass surgery?"

This book supplies the answer.

Coronary artery bypass grafting (CABG) is now one of the more commonly performed major operations in the United States. At the present time, 200,000 operations are performed each year, at an estimated cost of $4 billion—a substantial portion of the nation's total health-care expenditure. These figures do not include the numerous tests, including cardiac catheterization, by which patients are selected for the operation. Much controversy and confusion exists within the public and among many physicians about who should have the surgery and whether it does indeed save lives.

A 1983 survey by the National Heart, Lung and Blood Institute estimated that at least 15 percent of bypass surgeries are not needed. This study, called the Coronary Artery Surgery Study (CASS), conducted between August 1975 and May 1980, divided patients with coronary artery disease into those treated with surgery and those receiving medical treatment. The results of this important study, reported in 1983, found no significant difference in mortality at the end of five years between patients treated surgically or medically, except for certain specific circumstances. This study, which will be discussed later on, is the impetus for this book.

The true figure of the number of bypass operations that are not needed is probably higher. This is of very major concern to the five million Americans suffering from coronary artery disease. Five hundred fifty-five of these will die per year. As this is a serious operation that has risks and is very costly, patients and their families need guides to answer crucial questions: What is bypass surgery and the technique involved? What are the risks? What are the indications? If I am diagnosed as having angina, or have had a heart attack, should I undergo cardiac catherization to study my arteries and then have bypass surgery? *Should I get a second opinion?* (This last can be answered directly—and the answer applies to getting a second opinion on all major medical issues: "Yes. Yes. Yes.")

In this book, I will discuss alternatives to bypass surgery. In most cases these alternatives are as good, if not better, than the surgery. I will outline in specific detail when the test procedure called coronary angiography (X-ray of the coronary arteries) should be performed and when it can be delayed or omitted. Since its inception some fifteen years ago, coronary artery bypass surgery has given cardiologists a brilliant tool to treat coronary artery disease. But is it being overused?

A Coronary Tale

At the age of eight, James was a vigorous boy who made the most of his average scholastic ability. His father, Bill, a robust mechanic and a World War II veteran, smoked three packs of cigarettes a day, ate bacon and eggs for breakfast, and prided himself on being able to eat a gallon of ice cream at one clip.

James was slight in appearance and wished he had some more "fat" like his hero father. His mother encouraged him to drink a quart of milk per day and approved of the healthy appetite he displayed, devouring one cheeseburger after another. All the cheeseburgers, malted milkshakes, candy bars, and extra snacks did not fatten James.

One late afternoon after school, some of the boys met in an alley behind the movie theater. They purchased a pack of cigarettes and James coughed his head off with each puff. He hated that feeling, but he kept trying.

At the age of fifty, James's father, one morning after a big snowstorm, began to shovel the sidewalk. The morning air was refreshing, and if he could finish the steps before going to work, there would be less to do when he returned.

He began to shovel with a compulsive passion, his face becoming redder by the minute as the wind circled around his neck. Bent slightly forward, he made up his mind that he was going to lose weight because his huge belly was slowing him down. He was determined to return to his World War II size, an athletic body with not an ounce of fat.

As he was shoveling the snow, he felt a wave of nausea, and every time he bent down, heartburn. The night before he had had some kielbasa and several beers, as well as two slices of cream pie that his wife had baked. Beginning to burp a great deal, he decided to quit shoveling, take some bicarbonate of soda, and then go to work.

He felt unusually exhausted this particular morning, and as he walked into the kitchen, his wife remarked that his face had turned from pink to a kind of green.

"A little indigestion from your delicious cooking," he

replied. He reached into the cabinet, found the bicarbonate of soda, placed a tablespoon in his glass of water, swallowed it, and for a few minutes felt relieved. Then the heartburn returned with an intensity he had never felt before, and he began to perspire profusely. His wife, concerned, called the family doctor, who lived just a few blocks down the street.

Dr. B. came, examined him carefully, and advised Bill to go to bed, diagnosing an acute indigestion attack. "Maybe it's even your gallbladder," he said.

Bill went to bed, took out a cigarette, and began to smoke, but he did not feel better. Several hours later, the doctor was called again. Bill was now suffering from excruciating pain in his chest. The ambulance brought Bill to the hospital, and he was placed on a general medical floor (it was 1960, and the hospital had neither a coronary care unit nor an intensive care unit).

An electrocardiogram was taken at the bedside and indicated that Bill was probably having a heart attack. Morphine was given and he was placed in an oxygen tent. A priest was called (protocol in this hospital), and the last rites were given.

Throughout the night, the pain increased in severity. More morphine was given intravenously. By 4:00 A.M. his lungs were filling with fluid, and the doctors diagnosed Bill as having heart failure.

At 5:00, with a doctor at the bedside running the electrocardiogram, Bill's heart began to beat erratically. He continued to chat about his job during the entire time, even when his blood pressure was no longer measurable. At 7:00, his heart suddenly stopped and he was pronounced dead. Diagnosis: myocardial infarction, or heart attack.

James took his father's death badly. As the years passed, he more than fulfilled his wish of not being a skinny kid, and by the time he graduated from college, he was 5′8″ and weighed 270 pounds. Like his father, he smoked three packs of cigarettes a day.

James was honest, conscientious, and hardworking. When he started his job as a salesman for the B & B Corporation, he was earning a decent salary. By the time he was forty-nine, he was a regional manager, which required a great deal of traveling. When he was home on the weekends, it was hard for him to slow down. On a typical working day, at six o'clock in the morning he would listen to the news and then read the paper while on the toilet in order not to waste time. By 7:45 he would have finished reading the paper and would scramble up three eggs and cheese, which he gulped down with his coffee as if he was fearful that any minute some demon would snatch it all away. In his usual frenzy, he would drive his car to the railroad station to catch the 7:55 to the city.

There were two telephones on his desk, and at nine o'clock he would be talking to the salesman from Peoria, Illinois, holding the phone between his ear and his shoulder while writing his notes and puffing on his cigarette. Toward the end of the morning, he would have finished his fourth cup of coffee and tenth cigarette and experienced two loose bowel movements. James was a typical Type A person (to be discussed later).

He continued in this fashion until the age of fifty-four, when he began to complain of an enormous amount of fatigue.

"I'm getting older," he told his wife, "but I know I can't slow down. We have two boys in college, and we just put the addition on the house. I've got to make more money."

He developed a severe sleep disorder. By 9:00 most nights, totally exhausted, he fell asleep, but by one o'clock he was wide awake, his mind racing. His doctor gave him Valium and a sleeping pill, which helped him to get through the night, except that it made him feel like a zombie in the morning. The more exhausted he was, the more he smoked and the more alcohol he consumed. His sexual desire was waning and he was becoming increasingly irritable.

It was during an extraordinarily difficult week, after he returned from a sales meeting in San Diego, that he began to feel poorly. First, he noticed some funny tinglings in his chest, which he disregarded; then he felt some actual heaviness and tightness. It sometimes woke him up from a sound sleep.

In spite of James's extreme exhaustion, he still continued his frantic pace. His chest discomfort increased as the days went on, sometimes lasting five minutes, the pain going down his left arm and then disappearing.

"You should slow down," his wife told him one day when he returned from work. "You look gray. Maybe you need a vacation."

In the same breath she told James that they were going to spend a weekend in Vermont. But it was hardly restful. The martinis flowed like the Vermont mountain streams. On the way up to their cabin, they stopped in a grocery store to pick up cigarettes—five packs—and steaks. With all the alcohol, the freedom from his office, and the laughter, he paid little attention to the chest discomfort.

On Monday morning, he was up again at six, going through his usual routine of lighting up a cigarette, shaving, sitting on the toilet, and glancing at the *Wall Street Journal*, all at the same time. When he arrived at his office, he felt worse than he ever had felt in his life. Holding the phone to his ear, writing notes, and giving directions to his secretary, he called his family doctor, who insisted that he leave his desk and come immediately over to his office.

His physician took a thorough history and listened attentively to the story of his chest pain. After the history was taken, an examination disclosed that his blood pressure was 170/120, his pulse was beating furiously, and he was perspiring. His serum cholesterol, moverover, was a high 380, and his lung function was poor.

James's doctor told him that he was probably suffering from angina.

The following day, James had an exercise stress test performed, which confirmed the diagnosis. Several days later, he had a plastic tube placed into his heart so that the doctor could visualize the arteries. It was found that two of the major arteries were 75 percent narrowed. Several days later, James underwent a bypass operation, with the placement of two new blood vessels. (More about James later.)

Bill's story illustrates, in a general way, how coronary artery disease was managed in 1961—a far cry from the incredible technology available to his son in 1984. But could coronary artery bypass surgery have been avoided for James and could the results been just as good?

In the next few sections, in order to give the reader a greater understanding of what coronary artery bypass surgery is all about, I will describe some of the important basic concepts of coronary artery disease and what James could have done to avoid surgery.

Acknowledgments

For their expertise and their excellent advice I wish to thank Dr. Lawrence Cohen, Ebenezer K. Hunt Professor of Medicine, Yale University School of Medicine, and Dr. Kenneth Schwartz, Associate Clinical Professor, Yale University School of Medicine, and Chief of Cardiology, Griffin Hospital; and for all the sound advice on the manuscript, Dr. George Kraus, Director of Health, City of Milford, Connecticut, Lecturer in Public Health and Assistant Clinical Professor, Yale University School of Medicine. A special thanks to the nurses and staff of the Coronary Care Unit of the Yale-New Haven Hospital and the Hospital of St. Raphael. The idea for this book was suggested to me several years ago by Tom Wolf and the late Leslie Fairchild. I wish to thank my secretary, Madelyn Bartone, for the excellent typing, and my assistant, Karen Bowman, for the superb illustrations, and Leonard Kent, Professor of English, Quinnipiac College, for his excellent assistance.

I

HEART DISEASE AND HEART ATTACKS

1

Angina and Coronary Artery Disease

THE heart, thought by Aristotle to be the seat of the soul, pumps ten pints of blood through the body every day, supplying 300 trillion cells along a route of 75,000 miles. It lies behind the breastbone, in the center of the chest, somewhat to the left. Its apex, or narrow end, points downward. The heart is covered by a protective sac called the *pericardium.* If the heart becomes enlarged, it is displaced to the left and to the right, past the breastbone, as well as forwards and backwards. The heart is divided into the left and right sides and is about the size of a human fist, its weight ranging from approximately eight to fifteen ounces in a large man. The average length is about four inches.

The arteries that supply the muscle of the heart are called the *coronary arteries.* (See figure 1.) Two major ones arise from the aorta: a left coronary artery and a right coronary artery. The left main artery supplies the front of the heart, and the right artery supplies the back of the heart. After the left main artery leaves its origin, it immediately divides into branches, called the *left anterior descending artery* and the *circumflex.*

When the coronary arteries become narrowed, impeding the flow of blood and precious oxygen to the heart muscle, the condition is called *coronary artery disease.*

The classical symptom the patient feels when there is not enough blood and oxygen going through the arteries is chest pain called *angina* or *angina pectoris.* Angina that does not subside can mean a heart attack is in progress, but it is important to know that first, not all chest pain is angina, and second, the majority of people who experience angina do not die or suffer a heart attack.

The condition *arteriosclerosis* is commonly called "hardening of the arteries." Both terms indicate that the artery becomes thick and hard and loses its elasticity. *Atherosclerosis* is a form of arteriosclerosis in which the layers of the artery become thickened and irregular by deposits of cholesterol. These deposits narrow the arteries and impede the flow of blood, causing the symptom of chest pain, or angina pectoris, and eventually can lead to a heart attack. Throughout

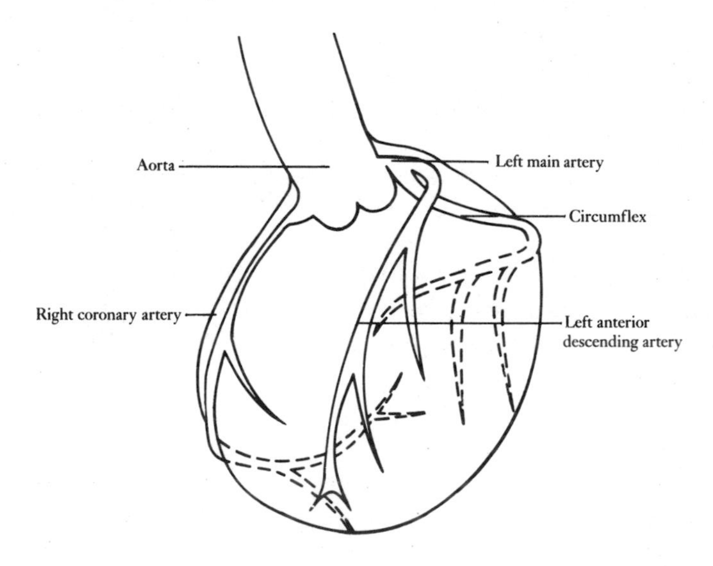

Figure 1. The coronary arteries

this book, I shall use the term atherosclerosis in referring to cholesterol deposits of the coronary arteries.

Angina, from the Latin, means strangulation. Angina is a sensation—a heaviness, a tightness—in the chest, usually felt over the breastbone or next to the breastbone, sometimes radiating down the left shoulder or spreading in fan fashion to the jaw. It is often accompanied by some sweating and apprehension; occasionally there is shortness of breath and anxiety about dying. It is a frightening and oppressive feeling that may last a few minutes and then disappear spontaneously, or remain. Some patients describe the sensation as "an elephant sitting on my chest." Other patients, with an anguished facial expression, may clench their fists on their chest because of severe pain.

The pain can be brought on by different things—exercise, anxiety, eating, change in temperature, drinking something cold—or by nothing at all. It can just as readily occur at rest, when a patient is sitting quietly in his chair, or fast asleep in his bed, as it can while he is playing tennis or having a fight with a spouse.

There are many faces of angina. For example, instead of a heaviness or a tightness in the chest, it may be felt as heartburn. (This does not mean that every heartburn is angina. Most heartburns are due to acid's flowing back into the esophagus.) Because the pain nerves of the heart fan out throughout the chest and even to the back, the pain of angina can also sometimes be felt distant from the heart. Not infrequently, the only symptom might be pain in the wrist or arm, or a pain in the upper back, which means that the back of the heart is suffering oxygen lack. Doctors call this *referred pain.*

Patients may complain of angina only when they are on vacation. Others have this frightening symptom only when they make love. Older cardiologists have described "week-end angina," "holiday angina," "mother-in-law angina," and "Monday night football angina." Typical angina symptoms can occur with normal coronary arteries in the presence of diseased valves. A critically narrowed aortic valve, called *aortic stenosis,* can cause angina.

By taking a careful history, performing a clinical examination, and administering appropriate tests, a firm diagnosis can usually be made. It is the responsibility of the physician to make the diagnosis of angina only after careful consideration and proper testing. Unfortunately, sometimes this diagnosis is made too hastily and the patient is led to believe he has a serious condition that he in fact does not have, resulting in undue hardship, fear, and changes in mode of living. There are a variety of other causes of chest pain, which I will discuss later in this chapter.

Telling a patient that he has angina immediately fills him with understandable but unnecessary fear. Atherosclerosis is no longer thought of as an illness with no treatment and no cure. Coronary artery disease is a progressive illness, but its progress may be halted and perhaps reversed.

Prior to 1980, physicians and patients had a somber view of this illness. Today, there are an estimated 5.4 million individuals who have been diagnosed as having coronary artery disease. Of these, 683,000 have been admitted to hospitals in the United States suffering an acute heart attack.

Heart attack, myocardial infarction, and *coronary thrombosis* mean the same thing. The blood ceases to flow through the coronary arteries because the artery is completely clogged by a clot, or thrombus, resulting in death of the muscle. The heart muscle suffers from oxygen hunger, and if the oxygen is not supplied, the heart muscle will die. It has been found that the heart muscle can survive with decreased oxygen for a period from forty minutes to six hours. This fact has important therapeutic consequences, to be discussed later on, regarding salvaging the heart muscle that is drained of oxygen.

Dr. William B. Kannell, director of the department of preventive medical epidemiology at the Boston University Medical Center, has been studying angina pectoris in Framingham, Massachusetts, over a twenty-year period. His statistics, reported in 1980, demonstrated that 6 percent of average adult males per year can expect to have a heart attack, with a death rate of 4 percent per year. In some patients, angina appears for a while and then disappears. Others suffer with angina all their lives. Dr. Paul Dudley White, the renowned cardiologist, himself a sufferer for decades, followed patients with angina who survived thirty years. Ironically, angina may disappear following a heart attack.

Heart failure should not be confused with heart attack, myocardial infarction, or coronary thrombosis. It means that the pumping action of the heart becomes impaired. The blood then backs up into the lungs, causing shortness of breath and swelling of ankles, or the symptoms of heart failure. Heart failure can occur as the result of a heart attack, a diseased valve, or a muscle that is destroyed by a virus or other causes.

Spasm of the Coronary Arteries

The current concept of coronary artery disease holds that angina can result not only from clogging of arteries but also from spasm of the arteries. Dr. Artilio Maseri, of Pisa, Italy, has demonstrated that arteries do go into spasm and can cause anginal pain, irregular heartbeats, and even sudden death. This confirming observation has resulted in a totally new and exciting field of treatment with a specialized group of drugs called *channel blockers,* which will be discussed in a later chapter.

Typically, the cardiologist suspects spasm of the coronary arteries when angina occurs while the person is sitting or lying quietly, in contrast to pain occurring during activity. When spasm rather than just blockage is responsible for angina, this is sometimes indicated by characteristic changes in the electrocardiogram.

Chest Pain Confused with Angina

Pain arising from the chest has so many causes that it can sometimes dumbfound the doctor. As mentioned earlier, normal coronary arteries and a diseased aortic valve can give the pain of angina. Chest pain that is not at all typical, however, of angina, sometimes is associated with prolapse of the mitral valve, with the gastrointestinal tract, or it can be musculoskeletal in origin.

PROLAPSE OF THE MITRAL VALVE

Prolapse of the mitral valve is a very common condition seen in millions of women (6 per cent of the female population) and also very common in men. This is a condition that results when the leaflets of the mitral valve bulge into one of the chambers like a hammock. Sometimes this causes a heart murmur and is associated with chest pain. The diagnosis is readily made by the sonar examination of the heart, to be discussed later on.

I have seen hundreds of patients with the diagnosis of prolapse of the mitral valve. Often, this condition may cause irregular heartbeats. The chest pain, however, at times needs to be differentiated from angina. Usually, prolapse of the mitral valve is not a serious condition, and it should not be of concern to persons who have it.

GASTROINTESTINAL DISEASE MIMICKING ANGINA

Gastrointestinal disease can be a common cause for chest pain. Gas forming in the intestines can be trapped in a small pocket that loops around to the back of the heart and causes that constant, nagging, sticking pain that makes the person think he is suffering from a heart attack. The symptom is often relieved by burping. A careful history will characterize the pain as sticking and sharp, underneath the breast, not at all like the pain of angina that I have described. This is where the practice of medicine becomes an art—sorting out the pain of angina from other kinds of chest pain. Modern technology and testing can free this person from going through each day with the mistaken fear of heart disease.

Sixty percent of chest pain not coming from the heart originates from the esophagus—the tube that leads from the mouth to the stomach. Pain arising from the esophagus is usually dull and continuous and often spreads to the back. It is worsened by bending or stooping or after eating certain foods. This pain may be a "heartburn" or a dull ache, even a tightness in the chest feeling like angina. But, reader beware! Not all heartburns come from the swallowing tube. Sometimes the heartburn may in fact be angina. Any heartburn in a patient over forty who has risk factors (smoking, hypertension, obesity, diabetes, family history of heart disease) should be fully investigated to be sure it is not springing from the heart.

A *GI series* (gastrointestinal X-ray) may demonstrate a sliding hiatal hernia (the stomach partially slips into the chest and acid regurgitates into the esophagus). A firm diagnosis of pain coming from the esophagus can be arrived at by special tests that will demonstrate whether or not the esophagus goes into spasm or acid flows from the stomach back into the esophagus. These tests are performed by placing a tube into the throat, down into the esophagus; the tube then measures the pressure and flow of acid. It is an uncomfortable test, but it is very helpful. These tests, if positive, will provoke pain in the chest similar to the pain of angina.

A diseased gallbladder can cause chest pain and angina-like symptoms. Usually, typical gallbladder symptoms consist of recurrent episodes of belching and bloating after meals, especially after fatty meals. Some chest pains can signal a diseased gallbladder, especially if associated with these symptoms. A simple sonar examination of the gallbladder can help make the diagnosis. The symptoms of belching and bloating and chest pain, however, can still represent heart disease.

MUSCULOSKELETAL PAIN CAUSING CHEST PAIN

Pain can arise from the back of the neck (cervical spine) and spread to the chest, brought on by physical effort. The pain can even spread down the left arm, like anginal pain. It is usually caused by a pinched nerve in the neck. It is a sharp pain, readily reproduced by bending or turning the neck.

Sometimes pain can arise from the ribs at the point they meet the breastbone *(costochondral junction).* This pain, called the *Tietze syndrome,* is often mistaken for a heart attack. It is caused by inflammation of the rib ends and can be reproduced by pressing on the rib articulation.

Oversized female breasts can bend the spine forward and cause a chronic nagging pain in the chest. Patients with arthritis often complain of chest pain, but it is generally sharp and pulling.

There are many more causes of chest pain, such as pleurisy, pulmonary embolism (clots to the lungs) and inflammation of the heart, which the doctor has to differentiate from angina.

2

Diagnosing Coronary Artery Disease

PRIOR to our sophisticated tests, the diagnosis of angina was made from the history alone. The purpose of performing the tests is to confirm the diagnosis and measure the severity of the disease and to eliminate the possibility of a wrong diagnosis.

The diagnosis of angina cannot always be based on an electrocardiogram. The electrocardiogram of a person with angina symptoms is normal more than 50 percent of the time. The electrocardiogram records the electrical activity arising from the body of the muscle of the heart, and if this muscle is injured, waves of injury appear. Angina occurs often with no permanent muscle injury.

The following tests are used to confirm the diagnosis of coronary artery disease: 1) the exercise stress test; 2) the thallium stress test; and 3) cardiac catheterization.

The Exercise Stress Test

As early as 1857, a physician by the name of Edward Smith started to use the treadmill for exercise testing. The current exercise stress test is an extension of the Master two-step test devised in the late 1940s by Dr. Arthur Master of New York.

Instead of climbing up a number of prescribed steps in a given period of time, the person rides a bicycle or runs on a treadmill. Leads are attached from the chest to the electrocardiogram, and while the patient's heart is stressed, an electrocardiographic reading is taken.

In a normal individual, as the pulse rate increases and the blood pressure rises, there are no abnormal changes on the electrocardiogram. Waves, called *S-T segment* and *T waves*, record the activity of the heart. A rise of the S-T segment from the baseline is abnormal, as is a fall below the baseline (which is measured in millimeters). (See figure 2.)

When the coronary arteries are narrowed by 75 percent, not enough blood-carrying oxygen arrives at the muscle, and the heart sends out signals on the electrocardiogram by either an elevation or depression of the S-T segment. Along with these electrical changes, anginal pain may appear, the

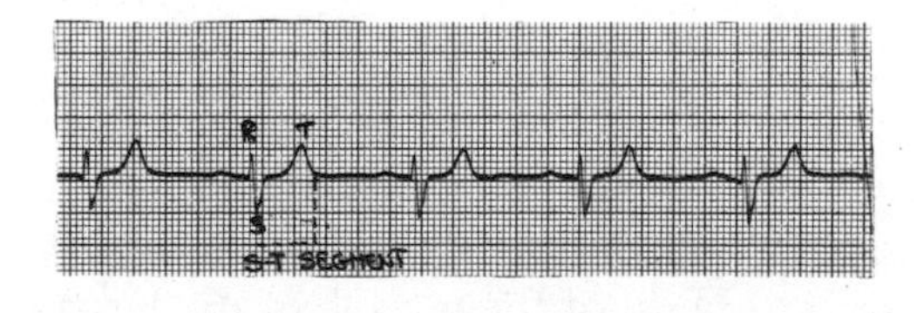

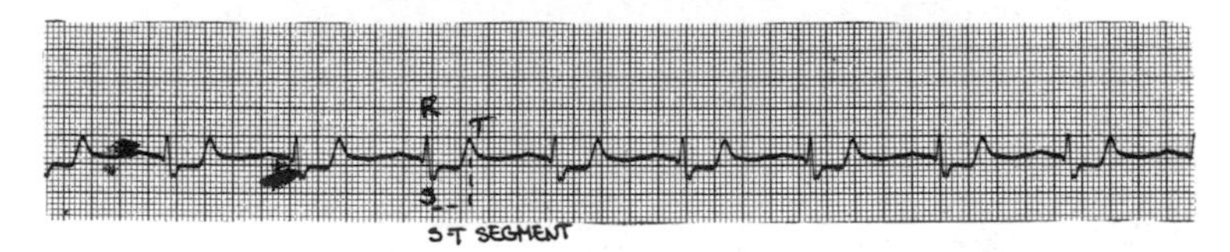

Figure 2. Electrocardiogram of stress test

blood pressure may drop, and sometimes the pulse may actually fall. These signs tell the doctor the test is positive. A slight change in the S-T segment is regarded as mildly abnormal, while a 3 mm or more drop is considered most abnormal, especially if there is accompanying chest pain.

According to the patient's age, a target goal in pulse rate is predetermined, and the patient is encouraged to achieve 85 percent of this target. For example, a fifty-year-old person, untrained, has a target heart rate of 180 so is encouraged to attain approximately 160 beats per minute. Often, the test is discontinued because of body fatigue; if the pulse rate has not been achieved, and if there are no changes, the test is considered non-diagnostic. On the other hand, if abnormal changes occur at a low pulse rate, the test is considered highly positive.

For persons who have a marked abnormal stress test, there is a 50 percent chance that their disease will progress in the next four to five years. Some patients may have an abnormal stress test and no heart disease, while others may have a normal stress test and have coronary artery disease. Patients with a normal stress may have disease of the tiny artery in the heart which is not registered by the stress test. This condition, sometimes called "small-vessel disease," calls for a further refinement of exercise stress testing, which will be described later on.

The physician performs the stress test using a set protocol prescribed by the American Heart Association. The physician must be in attendance along with the technician; the patient's pulse and blood pressure are carefully watched; and above all, the experienced physician will notice how the patient responds—his color, the expressions on his face—and will carefully monitor the electrocardiogram. A sudden pallor of face or a frightened look can alert the physician that something is about to happen—a precipitous drop in the blood pressure, or chest pain—and the test is discontinued.

The stress test should not be performed if the patient is having chest pain, as it can produce a full-blown heart attack. It should not be performed if the blood pressure is too high or if heart rhythm is irregular (if the heart is not contracting properly, the result is a slow rate, called *heart block*). Before the patient undergoes the test, an examination of the heart is necessary, as there are certain conditions that make it highly dangerous to have the test. For example, when the aortic valve is critically narrowed *(aortic stenosis)*, exercise can cause sudden death.

Rarely during the stress test does the patient suffer a heart attack. In one survey, a mortality rate of 10 per 150,000 was reported. All stress test laboratories are obliged to contain resuscitation equipment with trained personnel. Sometimes during the exercise, an abnormal heart rhythm can develop and the test is discontinued.

A test is considered grossly abnormal when the patient, at a low pulse rate, develops angina and the electrocardiogram turns very abnormal. This is called low-level test abnormality and tells the doctor that many of the blood vessels are afflicted, and that aggressive medical or perhaps even surgical treatment is in order.

There are many reasons other than heart disease why the electrocardiogram response can be abnormal during a stress test. An abnormal response can result from abnormality of the electrolytes in the blood, the medication that the patient is taking (for example, digitalis), or unknown reasons. Hyperventilation (when the patient breathes in and out rapidly) causes imbalances of the chemistry in the body and can make the electrocardiogram abnormal during a stress test.

I fully urge that a stress test be performed on patients over forty, whether they have risk factors (hypertension, smoking, family history of heart attack, and high cholesterol) or not, if they plan to undertake any exercise program, especially vigorous exercise programs like jogging, tennis, and racquetball that require a large expenditure of energy.

The purpose of the stress test is not only to determine if the patient has angina, but to identify people who are at risk of sudden death. It is a well-known phenomenon that certain patients, although they are clinically asymptomatic and may not have coronary artery disease, develop irregular rhythms that are forerunners of the fatal rhythm *(ventricular fibrillation)*. These arrhythmias sometimes can be identified with a properly conducted stress test. For example, some patients may develop an irregular rhythm and not be aware of it and their blood pressure may achieve dangerously high levels; these factors in themselves can bring on a heart attack or a stroke. Furthermore, some patients' cardiac reserves are so poor that the normal elevation of blood pressure and pulse that should follow exercise doesn't occur; the blood pressures may fall, and fainting episodes can result, and sometimes even sudden death. There are patients who have severe coronary disease who are totally symptom-free when performing physical effort but are prone to sudden death. Stress testing can identify these in at least two-thirds of the cases.

In a clinical setting the stress test is indispensable in detailing when angina arrives and at what level, and in informing the patient how much he can do with reasonable safety. An exercise prescription cannot be written intelligently unless one knows at what level the patient reaches his physiological capacity without apparent danger.

Unfortunately, the abuse of the stress test is legion. Many nonphysicians are performing this test for profit. Health clubs, health clinics, spas, and rehabilitation centers, not run by physicians, are capitalizing on our medical knowledge. A stress test should be performed only in the presence of a physician experienced in this procedure, in order to obtain a proper interpretation and for safety purposes.

Twenty-four-hour monitoring of the heart (using the Holter monitor) can sometimes reveal "silent coronary artery disease." It is called silent because there are ECG changes with no symptoms.

The Thallium Stress Test

The thallium stress is an expensive procedure but extraordinarily useful. By producing images of the heart muscle, it allows the physician to see indirectly how the blood circulates through the artery.

A radioisotope known as thallium is injected into the vein of the patient. The radioisotope is attracted to healthy tissue. It only lasts for a few hours and does not have any negative effects.

The patient runs on the treadmill or rides a bicycle. At the peak rate of his predicted heart rate, the thallium is injected into the vein. The patient lies down on the table and a special gamma camera scans the flow of thallium as it rushes to the heart muscle. If the heart muscle is not receiving enough blood, the thallium is not taken up by the heart.

The thallium stress test has an accuracy rate of finding coronary artery disease 90 percent of the time. Alas, as there still is a 10 percent or so chance that a patient with a normal thallium stress may be suffering from coronary artery disease, cardiac catheterization, to be discussed later, will be necessary to give the final answer to the question, "Do I have coronary artery disease?"

The stress test and the thallium stress test give us information regarding the circulation of the heart. Equally important to know is how efficient is the function of the heart. Does it contract well and pump blood to the rest of the body? Is the heart muscle injured because of not receiving enough blood?

An injured muscle that cannot pump efficiently (congestive heart failure) will cause blood to back up into the lungs, causing shortness of breath.

The Nuclear Scan

The state of the heart muscle—its efficiency—can be determined by the *nuclear scan*, or *MUGA (Multiple Gated Acquisition)*. In essence, the scan tells how the heart contracts. A radioisotope called thallium 201 is injected into an arm vein as the patient lies quietly on the examining table. A special camera takes pictures of the images formed of the contracting heart. The information is then fed automatically into a computer that reads out the percentage of efficiency, expressed as the *ejection fraction*. A 75 percent ejection fraction is considered excellent heart contractability and function and the patient has a good outlook, whereas an ejection fraction of 25 percent tells the physician the heart muscle is functioning poorly and the outlook is grim. With this low ejection fraction, something had better be done.

Sometimes classical angina can have an origin from a diseased valve, that is, a narrowed aortic valve *(aortic stenosis)*. It is imperative that this diagnosis be made, as angina arising from narrowing of the coronary artery is treated differently from angina arising from the aortic valve. Nitroglycerine, which is the workhorse medication for the treatment of angina, is not the drug to use for the treatment of aortic stenosis. The treatment of severe aortic stenosis includes the placement of a new artificial valve. This is one of the reasons that patients who have been diagnosed to have angina will also have a sonar examination, or echocardiogram, of the heart performed in order to check on the aortic and mitral valves.

The Echocardiogram

The sonar, or ultrasound, examination, cannot diagnose coronary artery disease. The sonar technique, which was used by the navy to detect submarines, is very useful to diagnose different forms of heart disease arising from the valve and the muscle, but is at its weakest in diagnosing arterial disease. The principle is to send soundwaves, coming from an electric crystal, to bounce off the heart; they are then placed into an electronic tube that converts them into an image. An actual true image of the movement of the heart and its valves is obtained. This is a test that is safe and can be repeated hundreds of times without any danger to the patient. The patient lies comfortably on an examining table, the technician places some special conduction paste on the chest (usually on the left side), and an instrument called a *transducer*, which is the size of a small cigar container, is rotated on the chest, sending out soundwaves toward the heart.

The Digital Angiogram

Other studies are on the horizon for visualization of the coronary arteries. One that is currently being evaluated is called *digital angiography*. In this technique, a catheter is placed into the vein and a dye is injected. As it travels through the arteries, a computer image is produced. It can give an overall picture of the coronary arteries, but it is not yet precise enough to determine severity of disease and the need for surgery.

Nuclear Magnetic Resonance

Nuclear magnetic resonance, or *NMR*, a technique which has been developed since 1940, has recently been used to examine the heart. This is a technique that does not involve any radiation; rather, it involves using the movement of molecules with the help of a magnet, an image being formed from the magnetic field. It has limited value in diagnosing disease of the coronary arteries, but it does visualize the actual heart muscle, which can tell us if the heart has been damaged.

All the tests described, and the clinical history, can give the physician strong evidence whether or not coronary artery disease is present, but in current clinical practice we still depend on the X-ray imaging of the artery, called *coronary angiography*, performed during cardiac catheterization—the gold standard of 1985.

Coronary Catheterization and Angiography

Cardiac catheterization means the passage of a tube through a blood vessel in the arm or thigh into the heart. When a dye is injected into the tube placed into the coronary artery and an X-ray is taken, it is called *coronary angiography*.

Any procedure has its risks and has to be weighed against the benefits. Cardiac catheterization gives us accurate information on whether or not the coronary arteries are diseased, or the valves are abnormal, or the heart is not functioning correctly.

In 1929, a German surgeon, Dr. Werner Forssmann, studying drawings on how tubes can be inserted into the veins of the heart of a horse, concluded that the same could be done to a man. Secretly, one afternoon, Dr. Forssmann injected a small amount of anesthetic into his arm and then proceeded to snake into a vein a long tube called a catheter, ordinarily used in the urinary tract. He was almost interrupted by a colleague, Peter Romas, who came storming into the room screaming, "What the hell are you doing?" Disregarding his colleague's plea, Forssmann placed a mirror in front of a fluoroscope screen and proceeded to snake the tube into his vein:

> I pushed the catheter in further, almost a two-foot mark. Now the mirror showed the catheter inside my heart with its tip in the right side ventricle. I had taken some X-rays for documentary purposes.

He was called insane by other physicians and was nearly fired from the Berlin Institute. But it was because of Dr. Forssmann's courageous experiment on himself that visualization of the coronary arteries (coronary angiography) is performed today. (He won a Nobel prize in medicine and physiology in 1956.)

Now that surgeons could see these arteries with their *lumen* (channels) obstructed, a logical sequence followed: bypass the obstruction and make new routes of flow to the sensitive heart muscle.

The number of cardiac catheterizations performed every year is approximately one-half million. It is an essential procedure before open-heart surgery, especially if the coronary arteries are going to be bypassed with new channels. There is practically unanimous agreement amongst cardiologists that cardiac catheterization and angiography should be performed in patients who have angina that does not respond to medical treatment and that makes the quality of life intolerable. It is also indicated if the cardiologist suspects that the main artery to the heart, the left main artery, is narrowed, which results in an annual death rate of 30 to 60 percent unless surgery corrects the abnormality. Cardiac catheterization will determine the extent of the narrowing of the coronary arteries and whether surgery will be able to correct it.

After a heart attack has occurred and the patient continues to have severe angina, it is wise to study his arteries. Some cardiologists feel that all patients who develop angina should have angiography in order to ascertain that serious disease is not missed. There are also occasions when the patient has typical chest pains, anginal in character, and yet the thallium stress is normal; these circumstances are an acceptable reason to perform angiography to make the diagnosis. I do not believe cardiac catheterization should be performed in a person who has an abnormal stress test but no symptoms of angina.

Cardiac catheterization should be performed (for angina)

1. if there is strong suspicion of left main artery disease;
2. if chest pain is severe and does not respond to medical treatment;
3. if the patient chooses to have surgery to treat his angina;
4. if chest pain continues after a heart attack;
5. if there is typical anginal pain, but only when the stress test and thallium stress test are normal;
6. if a very abnormal stress test is accompanied by chest pain;
7. if a stress test after a heart attack shows up very abnormal.

Cardiac catheterization can be delayed

1. if there is no chest pain, even if the electrocardiogram or the stress test is abnormal;
2. if the angina is mild and responds readily to medications;
3. if the patient decides not to have surgery;
4. if its aim is to prove the diagnosis of angina (especially if the thallium stress is abnormal);
5. if the goal is simply to study the arteries after a heart attack (if there are no further symptoms);
6. if there is an abnormal heart rhythm but no chest pain;
7. if there is an abnormal electrocardiogram during a routine physical;
8. if there is a heart murmur—mitral stenosis—that can be diagnosed with sonar waves.

Because James, whom we met in the introduction, had severe pain during his stress test, with serious electrocardiographic changes (S-T segment depression), he was advised to have a cardiac catheterization. The doctor explained to him how the procedure was going to be done:

"You will be admitted to the hospital the day before. A chest X-ray, an electrocardiogram, and blood tests will be done. A consent form will have to be signed indicating that you understand what the procedure is going to involve. The tube, which is called a catheter, will be inserted either in the right groin, or perhaps in the right arm. If you're going to be scheduled for the early hours in the morning, breakfast will be omitted, or if it's at a later time, a light breakfast may be given.

Cardiac catheterization is generally done in the X-ray department and lasts for about two hours. The test is performed by a highly specialized, trained physician with a team of other doctors and nurses. This is a safe procedure, and the death rate is very low, in the proximity of 0.2 percent. It is not a very comfortable procedure, but there is no need to be frightened, as all the people who are going to be involved are experts. There may be some pain and discomfort, and tingling feelings from the local anesthetic that is placed around the vessel where the tube is going to be placed. You may feel that your heart skips beats, and some palpitations may occur. I am going to give you some of the complications which can happen, but they are very rare."

One study disclosed a 3 percent complication rate. Some complications are extra-ordinarily rare. The catheter may accidentally perforate the heart, but generally this does not cause serious problems. There may be bleeding, with clotting of the artery; sometimes patients develop a stroke and a heart attack. A complication that tends to be a little more common occurs at the place where the catheter or tube is placed into the artery of the arm or leg; the incision can cause permanent damage by plugging the artery, because the wall gets slightly damaged from the catheter.

Allergies to the dye have also occurred. If the patient has any allergies, the doctor does a skin test first. It will generally be necessary for the patient to stay in the hospital overnight to be certain that none of these complications has occurred.

The cardiac catheterization laboratory is an amazing achievement of modern medicine. The setting is akin to a science fiction movie. The "cath team" is dressed in heavy lead-shield aprons with surgical masks and gowns. They work amidst X-ray equipment, monitoring screens, TV cameras, computers, and tables with strange-looking instruments, which surround the electric table on which the patient lies. Concerts of sounds—the beeping heart monitor and computers intermingling with the hissing sounds of oxygen—suffuse the room.

The doctor makes a small incision, one-quarter to one-half inch long, either in the right arm or right groin after it has been anesthesized with Novocain. There is a burning sensation when the Novocain is first injected. The patient should tell the doctor if there is any pain at all. He will be rotated from time to time on the table to get the proper angle for the photographs that will be taken, which will give some relief from lying motionless. He should not be frightened by the sounds and by such language as "give another puff" or "he has a PVC." PVC, for example, simply means preventricular contraction—an extra beat.

As the dye is injected into the heart, the patient may feel a hot sensation traveling from the top of his head to the tips of his toes. As the dye goes into the arteries, the doctor will ask him to cough to force the dye back out. Then the catheter will be removed and firm pressure will be applied to the place of insertion with a large pressure bandage. For several hours after that, he will be asked to lie quietly to prevent any bleeding. Coughing or sneezing should not make him anxious about anything being dislodged. Just applying the hand over the bandage will help prevent any bleeding.

James agreed to undergo cardiac catheterization after he understood all the benefits and possible complications. The procedure was uneventful. He returned to his room after one to one and a half hours, and he was discharged from the hospital the following day. At a cardiac catheterization conference, his case was presented to numerous cardiologists and it was concluded that two of his vessels were 85 percent obstructed. It was the opinion of his own cardiologist that he would benefit from having coronary artery bypass surgery; others disagreed.

James was now given a choice of surgery or medical treatment. He was told, in 1982, that if one vessel is critically narrowed, the death rate per year is in the vicinity of 4 percent without surgery; if two vessels are diseased, as was his case, that death rate is between 7 and 10 percent, and if three vessels are diseased, the mortality rate without surgery increases markedly in a five-year period—up to 50 percent.

The doctor explained to him that the angina occurs when the degree of arterial narrowing is greater than 90 percent; however, a 75 percent reduction can also cause angina if the person is exercising or walking briskly. If the heartbeat suddenly increases, as during intercourse or exercise, angina can also occur. Some patients may suffer no angina at all, even with critical narrowing of the arteries, but may sustain a heart attack, referred to sometimes as a silent heart attack. That was the state of the art in 1982. However, in 1984, the Coronary Artery Surgery Study revealed that the annual mortality rate for people with one diseased vessel, treated medically, was 1.4 percent; for two vessels, 1.2 percent; and three vessels, 2.1 percent.

James did have an alternative to surgery, because his life expectancy would be the same with surgery or not. Today, if James was confronted with the decision whether or not to undergo coronary arteriography, he probably would have declined to do so, as his symptoms were minimal. A thorough trial of medical treatment would have been prescribed, and then, if he did not respond, surgery would have been recommended. If he did decide to have coronary arteriography, he also would have available to him another recent alternative to bypass surgery, angioplasty.

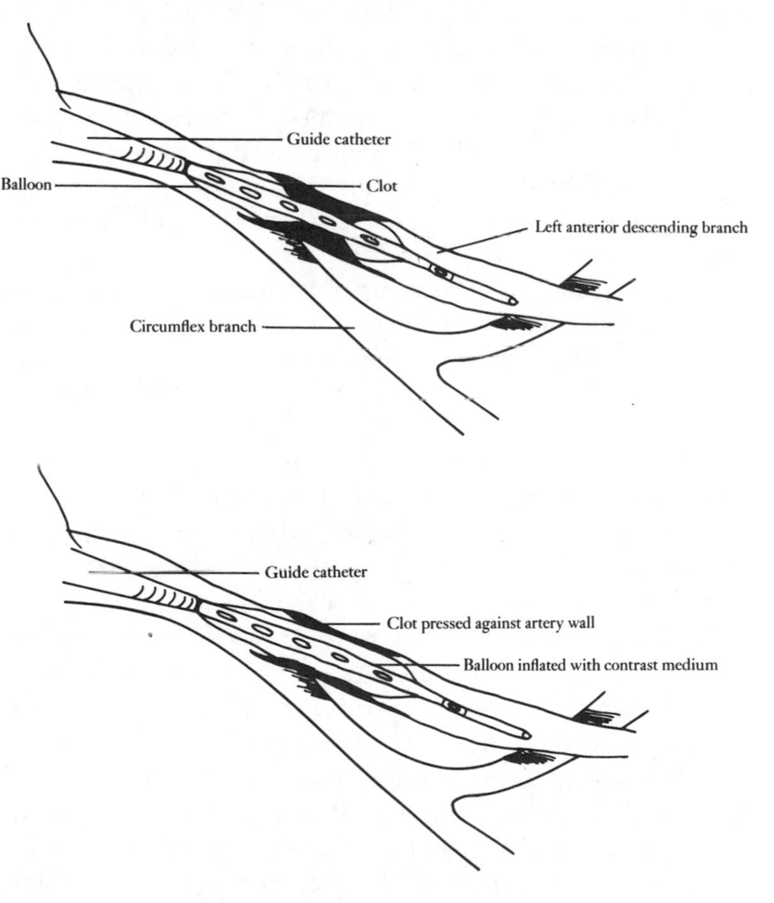

Figure 3. Coronary angioplasty

Angioplasty

Drs. Charles T. Dotter and Melvin P. Jukins were confronted with blocked arteries in an eighty-two-year-old woman with gangrene. These doctors snaked a catheter through the artery and pressed the clot against the wall, which resulted in opening the artery. In 1977, the technique was applied to coronary arteries, at the Zurich Medical College in Switzerland, by Dr. Andres Gruntzig. The catheter is introduced into the artery of the arm or leg and guided along in the same way as during cardiac catheterization. A tiny uninflated balloon, a small tube, is threaded through this larger catheter and is placed along the atherosclerotic plaque. The balloon is inflated for several seconds, flattening the cholesterol plaque against the arterial walls, and the passage is opened.

It is successful in 85 percent of patients, or more; it unblocks the arteries 90 percent of the time tried; however, in 20 percent of patients, the artery can block again within two months. The person who plans to undergo this procedure must be ready to also have bypass surgery in case of failure.

The indications for angioplasty are, in many ways, the same ones as for bypass surgery. It is presently being tried when more than one artery is blocked. The procedure takes about two hours. Dye is injected after the procedure to be certain that the artery is not blocked. Then the patient is returned to the coronary care unit for careful monitoring of his heart and blood pressure. As in cardiac catheterization, the patient will be instructed to avoid any movement of the leg in which the tube had been inserted. Bed rest should continue for up to two days. Often, after the angiography, a stress test is performed to check if the artery has remained open. Some cardiologists feel that 10 percent or more of patients who have coronary artery disease may be candidates for this procedure. Up to the present time, several thousand patients have undergone this new technique. A registry was established in 1979, called the Percutaneous Transluminal Coronary Angiography, or PTCA, at the offices of the National Institutes of Health. Thus far, a profile of patients reveals their mean age to be fifty-one and the duration of their angina to have been several months. Seventy-eight percent had disease in one vessel, 19 percent had two or three vessels involved, 2 percent had the left main artery closed. Ninety-five percent of all the patients who have had this procedure had symptomatic chest pain less than one month after the procedure.

The procedure failed either for technical reasons or because the blockage was too tight for the catheter to pass through. Approximately 7 percent of the patients had to have emergency bypass surgery. Death was reported in 1 percent. In due time, we will learn if this procedure can be used on an even wider basis. It has also been performed on people who have had bypass surgery and subsequently had their grafts close. Some of the complications recorded include heart attacks, hemorrhages, perforations, and infections.

A forty-nine-year-old athlete, who had a long family history of coronary artery disease and heart attacks, developed severe chest pain one day, after he finished playing tennis. Shortly afterwards, he fainted and collapsed on the floor. He was admitted to the coronary care unit, where the electrocardiogram determined that he had suffered an anterior wall infarction, a heart attack of the front wall of the heart. His pain was continuing after he had been in the unit for three hours. He received I.V. nitroglycerine, beta-blockers, channel calcium blockers—all with little response. His blood pressure began to drop and the doctors feared that death was imminent.

An emergency cardiac catheterization disclosed that the

left anterior descending artery was 98 percent blocked. During the cardiac catheterization, a balloon was inserted and compressed the plaque. The chest pain swiftly disappeared, the artery was unblocked, and the electrocardiogram improved. Ten days later, the patient left the hospital, no longer having chest pain. This patient fulfilled all the criteria for this procedure. He had severe intractable pain that was not relieved by intravenous nitroglycerine, and a small segment of the artery was narrowed. The entire procedure took approximately two hours in the cardiac catheterization laboratory, and the patient did not have to have open-heart surgery. He was an ideal candidate because the lesion was not yet too hard and calcified, and it was easy to compress.

Angioplasty is also now being used if more than one coronary artery is blocked, providing the obstruction is located in an area that is amenable to the balloon flattening procedure. As noted, it is also currently used for patients who have had bypass surgery and have had the grafts close.

Medicine is forever on the move. It is dynamic, and if we recommend a procedure at a particular time and place, it does not necessarily mean that we will recommend it several years later.

3

The Heart Attack

THE first sign of having clogged arteries may be a heart attack, or the attack may have been preceded by angina for a considerable number of years. On the other hand, the first sign of having coronary artery disease could be sudden death. A heart attack can occur as the result of spasm of the coronary arteries. Heart attacks can occur when a partially clogged artery suddenly becomes completely closed and is unable to deliver any oxygen to the heart. If the heart suffers from oxygen deprivation, it is called *ischemia*, or *ischemic heart disease.* When the heart muscle is partially destroyed, the term myocardial infarction is used.

Patients suffering from angina which does not get relieved in fifteen to twenty minutes need to be transported immediately to the emergency room because they may be having a heart attack. The pain is sudden, severe, prolonged, usually located in the region of the chest or upper part of the abdomen. The victim may be stricken while at rest or at work, when awake or asleep—sometimes without any warning. It may begin as a relatively mild persistent discomfort which becomes increasingly severe; or it may strike with a sudden, terrifying, severe intensity. The pain has been described as a constriction, an oppression, a compression, a sensation similar to the pain of acute angina pectoris. It is more crushing in intensity than angina and becomes, sometimes, completely unbearable. It can be a choking, vise-like, heavy feeling, or stabbing, dull, boring, or burning in quality. The pain may sometimes feel like severe indigestion or heartburn. (In fact, years ago, in the obituary pages, a patient's death was sometimes described as, "He died of acute indigestion.")

The pain is usually located behind the breastbone (sternum), spreading to both the front and back of the chest, down the left arm, and down to the abdomen. Sometimes it radiates to the jaw, to the neck, and to the teeth, persisting for an hour or more. The pain may be intense, then disappear entirely, and then reappear again for one or two hours. More often than not, it is accompanied by marked perspiration and fear. The patient may feel weak, dizzy, and nauseous, and may actually vomit. Sometimes he may feel a great deal of thirst. Unfortunately, many times, the patient may procrastinate about his symptoms and try to walk them off, or alleviate them by taking a hot bath, lying down, or taking a shot of whiskey or an antacid. Often the victim interprets the pain as an attack of indigestion or muscle shoulder pain and does not seek any help. Sometimes the pain may be of such mild intensity that the patient forgets about the pain entirely, and only after seeing a physician a week or more later, the electrocardiogram disclosing that myocardial infarction had occurred, does he realize he's had a heart attack.

The appearance of the patient sometimes is classic. Sitting or lying down, he is apprehensive, with eyes bulging, drenched in sweat, with marked weakness, nauseated, sometimes vomiting, feeling anxious and fearful of impending death. He may be sitting, clenching his fists against his chest. He may tear or clutch at his chest to remove a weight or release a vise-like pain. He may massage it vigorously as one does a cramp in the leg, thrashing from side to side, crouching and lying on the floor, or raise his hand above his head, lying in bed clutching at the head of the bedstead. If the blood pressure suddenly falls and he goes into shock, he may become confused, develop an ashen color, lips and fingers becoming blue; his hands and feet and the tip of his nose become cold and moist, and there may be a mottled bluish appearance of the skin.

When the left coronary artery is completely clogged, destruction of the front of the heart occurs. This is called an *anterior wall infarction.* If the right coronary artery is blocked, the back and the lower portion of the heart may be destroyed; this is called an *inferior wall infarction.* Both types of infarction sometimes occur together.

Dr. James Herrick, in 1912, described the different patterns of what happens in heart attacks. It was through the work of Dr. Samuel Levine and Dr. Paul Dudley White, as noted, that we first learned the details of a myocardial infarction, in 1929.

Atypical location of heart attack pain may occur: severe prolonged pain in the shoulder, in the wrist, in the elbow, neck, teeth, back, or abdomen. In contrast to the pain of angina, it is of long duration. Repeated doses of morphine are sometimes needed to relieve the pain. The patient may have difficulty breathing. The breathing difficulty results from the heart's not being able to pump properly and the blood's backing up into the lungs. This situation is called *pulmonary edema.*

Case: A fifty-one-year-old male who was a heavy smoker had just returned from a baseball game with his family. After the Red Sox won the game, the man took his wife to a pizza parlor and finished off two pizzas. Driving back home, he experienced severe heartburn, which did not subside. He began to perspire and his wife administered an antacid, which gave him some relief. The heartburn, however, persisted and they decided to immediately stop in at an emergency room. An electrocardiogram displayed the typical changes of a heart attack. The patient had an excellent recovery two weeks later. Delayed medical care for a heart attack can be disastrous.

Case: A gentleman, fifty-four years old, was on vacation, and each morning he took his regular walk into the forest before his family awoke. On this particular morning, after breakfast, he started his walk and began to feel ill. He sat down, nauseated, and began to perspire. After resting a few minutes, he continued his walk, burped, and was feeling somewhat relieved. By the time he arrived back home, he was gray in appearance and he was perspiring. His wife became frightened.

"I'm fine," he said. "It's only indigestion."

His wife insisted that they drive to the local emergency room. An alert intern took a careful history and discovered that the doctor had been having "heartburn" for several months. An electrocardiogram was taken which disclosed that he had had a massive myocardial infarction involving both the front and back of his heart. Almost six hours had passed from the time that the patient felt ill to the time of his admission into the hospital. Unfortunately, an hour after he arrived in the emergency room, he went into cardiac arrest and was unable to be resuscitated.

Comment: This sad case tells us two things: the heart attack presented with gastrointestinal symptoms, the gentleman was self-diagnosing himself as having indigestion. Obviously, delay in receiving care for a myocardial infarction can be disastrous. More lives would be saved if patients sought earlier medical attention.

Case: A forty-nine-year-old insurance salesman was playing tennis. After a vigorous game, he and his tennis partner sat drinking cold beer. Shortly after, he began to complain of severe pain in his wrist. His tennis partner advised him to place ice on the wrist and perhaps take a few Bufferin. The tennis player, when he returned home, felt extraordinarily exhausted and began to perspire. At the insistence of his wife, he was brought to the emergency room, where his appearance was gray and his pulse thin and feeble (thready); his blood pressure was barely obtainable. An electrocardiogram was taken, which disclosed he had suffered a heart attack in the back of his heart. His physical condition was excellent prior to the heart attack. He survived his attack and was completely rehabilitated. He still plays tennis.

Case: An obese fifty-eight-year-old traveling salesman had excruciating pain in his back, so severe that he began to perspire, and he drove his car directly to the emergency room. He had a long history of hypertension, heavy cigarette smoking, alcohol abuse, and severe overeating. The doctor on call discovered that the pain actually had also been felt in the front of the chest but was predominantly located in the upper portion of his back. The physical examination disclosed a man with a blood pressure of 220/120 and a pulse of 100, who was perspiring profusely and had an agonized look on his face. Morphine sulphate was given for his pain. An electrocardiogram showed that he had sustained a heart attack in the back portion of his heart. The patient ws treated in the coronary care unit and survived his initial heart attack.

Comment: In patients having heart attacks, the nerve fibers may send out messages of pain to the back. Most of the time, this is not the presentation of a heart attack, but it does, clearly, occur.

Treatment

Prior to 1960, patients admitted with a heart attack had a 40 percent chance of dying during their hospitalization. At that time, they would be placed in a general medical ward and enclosed in bulky plastic oxygen tents with no monitoring equipment. We knew little of resuscitation when cardiac arrests occurred.

As early as 1939, Dr. Claude Beck, who had learned from Dr. John Hooker in 1933 that animals could be resuscitated by mechanical massaging of the heart, recommended that hospitals have resuscitation squads. In 1956, a sixty-five-year-old man suddenly developed a chaotic heartbeat (ventricular fibrillation). The man was rushed to the operating room, his chest was opened by Dr. Beck, and cardiac massage was performed. An AC current was administered to the fibrillating heart, and the patient was successfully resuscitated. From then on it was not uncommon for patients' chests to be opened and internal cardiac massage to be performed.

Also in 1956, Dr. Paul Zoll and his associates devised a defibrillator, which sent electrical shocks through the chest wall, and emergency rooms were then equipped with this bulky equipment. Through the work of Dr. William Louwenhoven, doctors learned that the heart could be effectively massaged without opening the chest, and that circulation could be maintained if the massaging was accompanied by mouth-to-mouth resuscitation. Dr. H. W. Day, at the Bethany Hospital in Kansas City, organized a mobile crash cart, equipped with a defibrillator and external pacemaker to get the heart beating again. The trained team responded to a code signal whenever a cardiac arrest occurred anywhere in the hospital. Unfortunately, pushing the clumsy equipment took the team too long to arrive at the scene, and heart patients were soon placed in a designated area.

On May Day, 1962, an eleven-bed intensive care unit was opened in Kansas City. In 1962, the elaborate modern equipment included machinery that could measure blood pressure, respiration, and temperature; there were also cardiac monitors. The doctors soon realized that 95 percent of patients admitted into a coronary care unit developed an irregular heartbeat (arrhythmia), with 50 percent involving potentially serious consequences. Today, arrhythmias are swiftly recognized and treated, and this is no longer a major cause of death.

Today, once the patient has arrived in the coronary care unit, there is more than an 85 percent chance of survival. It is estimated that over a million patients are hospitalized each year with a heart attack. Patients who do not have any complications can be discharged from the hospital within a five- to ten-day period. Women who have sustained heart attacks have more serious advanced arteriosclerosis, for reasons yet to be learned. Women also have a higher death rate than men, as do patients over the age of seventy, who have a three to four times greater death risk than those sixty-nine years old or less. Those patients who have a large anterior wall infarction are at the highest risk of dying. Most deaths, about two-thirds of them, occur outside of the hospital within the first hour after the onset of chest pain.

A recent study, called the Australian Perth Coronary Register, recognized that among patients who had suffered a heart attack, those with the worst survival rate were: 1. smokers; 2. those who were suffering from hypertension and diabetes; 3. older patients; and 4. those who had previous heart attacks.

Once the patient is placed in the coronary care unit, he receives morphine for pain and oxygen is administered through nasal prongs. After a day or two, if the patient remains well, he is moved from the coronary care unit to a step-down unit and a rehabilitation program is started. At the end of one week to ten days, all going well, the patient is discharged.

Dr. Thomas Killip has classified the severity and prognosis of a heart attack according to the following:

Class 1—no heart failure and no complication rate: a mortality rate of 6 percent;

Class 2—mild to moderate heart failure: a mortality rate of 17 percent;

Class 3—serious heart failure with pulmonary edema: a mortality rate of 38 percent;

Class 4—shock: a mortality rate between 81 and 95 percent.

The definitive diagnosis of having sustained a myocardial infarction depends on the electrocardiographic changes and testing the blood for an enzyme called *creatine-phosphokinase*, or *CPK*. This enzyme is found throughout the body and in muscles, but there is a specific portion arising from heart muscle, called the *MB portion*. If the MB portion is elevated, then a heart attack has occurred. This test is performed early in the course of a heart attack; otherwise, the rise of the enzyme can be missed in the ensuing days.

The Framingham study has demonstrated that in the first year patients have a 15 percent chance of dying of their heart attack, the greatest risk occurring during the first six months. After one year, the annual death rate among former cardiac victims is approximately 5 percent, or less. Seventy-five percent of deaths are sudden and are due to an irregular heart rhythm. These figures are based on studies made before the use of new medications such as beta-blockers and channel blockers and may be altered by bypass surgery.

The cause of death is that so much of the heart muscle is destroyed that it is unable to sustain life. Different experiments have been tried to salvage the dying heart muscle. In the past, the infusion of sugar, water, and insulin has been advocated by some physicians. In a recent article in the *New England Journal of Medicine* (May 1984), it was affirmed that the major cause of death of the heart muscle is a clot (thrombus) in the artery, accompanied by spasm.

Patients in the coronary care unit who continue to have chest pain are given intravenous nitroglycerine. Years ago, doctors were taught never to give nitroglycerine during a heart attack because it was thought it might cause the blood pressure to drop and result in death. It was discovered, however, that nitroglycerine opens the arteries and can actually limit the extent of the destruction of heart muscle. Current investigations have also revealed that the use of beta-blockers and calcium channel blockers may limit the magnitude of a heart attack.

When the myocardial infarction is complicated by continual chest pain, drop in blood pressure, and accumulation of water in the lungs (heart failure), it is now common practice to thread a balloon-tipped catheter into the vein of the arm or thigh, or sometimes in the neck toward the pulmonary artery. This catheter enables doctors to measure effectively the various pressures in the heart and to see how the heart is working; and it gives them a guide concerning the medications and fluids to be administered. Occasionally, as sometimes happens during the course of a heart attack, the fluid in the body may actually drop and more fluid is needed to maintain a blood pressure.

Would it not be ideal if the clot in the coronary artery could be dissolved? For decades, scientists have been trying to prevent clots from forming in the heart and to dissolve the clots that do form. The body has a natural mechanism for the prevention of the clotting of blood as it circulates through millions of miles of channels. Unfortunately, there are times when the blood does clot when we do not want it to, especially within the coronary arteries. The clotting mechanism is a highly complicated process that involves various elements of the blood, among them platelets. The platelets tend to stick together, like chewing gum on a finger, and they clump and set up a series of events that cause the clot. The clot consists of a package of red cells and white cells and various tissues and platelets. In time, the clot becomes softer and holes form through it (recanalization), and the blood can then seep through. The clot should not be mistaken for the atherosclerotic plaque. The atherosclerotic, or cholesterol, plaque is a piling up of fatty materials and fibrous tissue. The thrombus can form on top of this plaque.

Since 1938, scientists have been trying to find a way to prevent the extension of a thrombus by the use of medications. *Heparin* was the drug used by Dr. Charles Best. It was discovered that certain animal tissues contain substances for the prevention of clotting of blood. *Hirudin*, a glandular secretion of leeches, is an anti-coagulant. A medical student by the name of J. McClean, then a sophomore at Johns Hopkins, isolated an anti-coagulant material from the heart and liver. Working in Dr. W.H. Howe's laboratory, he refined the material and called it *heparin*. Heparin was used for the purpose of dissolving clots for the first time in 1946, at the Karolinska Institute of Stockholm. We presently use Heparin routinely in small doses in every patient admitted to the coronary care unit, to prevent clots in the veins, which can break off and cause an *embolus*. An embolus is a blood clot or other substance, such as fat, air, or tumor, that travels in the bloodstream to a smaller vessel and causes obstruction to the flow of blood.

Another medication used for the prevention of clots is *coumadin*. Its discovery is an intriguing story. In the winter of 1922, veterinarians in the province of Alberta, Canada, and simultaneously in North Dakota, reported a bleeding condition in cattle. This illness was characterized by massive bleeding from minor injuries. The animals bled after just brushing against a tree. Because of the great economic loss, research was immediately begun by Dr. R. Schofield. He discovered that there was a poison in the spoiled sweet clover hay that the cattle ate and he was able to produce bleeding symptoms by feeding rabbits with it. These experiments continued through the years, and finally, in 1941, Dr. K.P. Link isolated and identified *Dicumarol* (coumadin). The first human experiments were successfully concluded at the Mayo Clinic.

Coumadin is an effective medication to prevent the extension of a clot once it has formed, and it also prevents the forming of clots, but it does not dissolve the clot. Nature dissolves the clot by enzyme systems within the body itself. Both of these drugs are continuously being used in the coronary care unit and after valve surgery, with the hope of preventing the formation of clots.

Low-dosage aspirin is reported to prevent a clot in the coronary artery. Currently, it is used in the setting of the coronary care unit when chest pain persists (unstable angina). One recent study demonstrated a 43 percent reduction in the death rate when aspirin is administered during the chest pain. In 1985, in some centers, patients having continual chest pain during a heart attack are given I.V. nitroglycerine, channel calcium blockers, and Heparin in order to slow down the clot that may be forming in the coronary artery.

Other researchers were now looking for a natural substance that would dissolve clots, and Dr. Sol Sherry, a pioneer in this work, has used an enzyme in urine, called *urokinase,* that can dissolve clots in veins by activating other chemicals. In the early years of his work, in Philadelphia, tons of urine had to be distilled to produce this product, and it has been said that on Monday mornings, volunteers had to carry gallons of urine into Dr. Sherry's laboratory.

A similar type of substance, *streptokinase,* was manufactured from the streptococcus microbe. Injection of streptokinase directly into the coronary arteries dissolves the clot and allows the flow of blood to proceed. Streptokinase is injected during cardiac catheterization. It is essential that this is done as swiftly as possible, within the first six hours of a heart attack; otherwise the clot may already have formed and caused the heart muscle to be destroyed. Streptokinase can also be given by intravenous infusion without the necessity of going into the coronary arteries. Some scientists, however, report that this method is less effective. It has not yet been fully established whether streptokinase changes the death rate of heart attack. The drug is currently being used in various medical centers and hospitals. A number of champions of this procedure, such as Dr. William Ganz, feel that the intravenous route is just as effective as the cardiac catheterization route.

Angiograms taken before and after streptokinase show the flow of blood right after the procedure. Some cardiologists, after an infusion of streptokinase, use the balloon catheter to widen the artery mechanically. Streptokinase, unfortunately, is not a selective chemical and can cause hemorrhage in other parts of the body.

Case: A fifty-three-year-old male had severe chest pain and there were changes on the electrocardiogram that made it certain a heart attack was in progress. The pain lasted for one hour, and three hours later streptokinase was infused into the left anterior descending artery. The clot disappeared, the pain subsided, and the patient was discharged pain-free, with minimal damage to his heart muscle. How long the artery will remain clot-free is unknown.

Other patients with similar history are not as lucky and do develop a heart attack. Some studies report a 70 to 80 percent success rate. The effectiveness of this form of treatment remains to be proven in the years ahead.

An exciting new discovery is the use of a clot dissolver (a *plasminogen activator*). It has a direct action on the coronary artery thrombosis and does not affect the rest of the clotting mechanism, as streptokinase does. Scientists are now looking to make this available for general use. It can be given intravenously, and in contrast to streptokinase, causes less overall reactions and bleeding. It is a natural substance found in our bodies.

The *tissue plasminogen activator* (TPA) may someday save patients from bypass surgery. It disappears from the blood in thirty minutes, and all clots in the arteries can be dissolved in less than two hours, saving most of the heart muscle from destruction. In the future, it may even be possible for patients to inject themselves at the first sign of a heart attack. At the present time, TPA is obtained from cultured human cells. (Interestingly, cancer cells also form a great deal of this substance.) Dr. Burton Sobel, of Washington University, and Dr. Colen Desire, of the University of Leuven in Belgium, among others, are presently working on this project.

Another new-frontier experiment is dissolving clots with laser beams. The laser has been used in eye surgery as a scalpel to cut away tissues. Preliminary results with different types of lasers are exciting. Dr. Dean Mason and his colleagues found that the laser beam can improve the opening of a blood vessel crowded with fibrous lipid and calcified obstructions. Some studies have already been performed on human beings in the University of Toulouse Medical School in France. Five patients who were about to undergo bypass grafting were instead treated with the laser. Their occlusion was reduced, and three weeks later, repeat angiography showed them still to be open.

We can look forward to the time when laser angioplasty will clean out our coronary arteries. At the present time, more work has to be done in order to keep the beam within distance of the artery, because complications have occurred. This procedure has not been approved by the FDA in our country. Most of the experimental work is currently being done on animals by a Stanford University team. The laser will reach the arteriosclerotic arteries through the standard catheters now used.

In many medical centers, during the course of a heart attack, patients who continue to have chest pain in spite of I.V. nitroglycerine, beta-blockers, channel blockers, and aspirin undergo cardiac catheterization. The clogged arteries are identified and are flattened out with a balloon *(balloon angioplasty).*

Before Discharge after a Heart Attack

Fifteen percent of the patients, the so-called high-risk patients, have a mortality range from 20 to 40 percent in the first year after discharge. These patients are identified as having frequent irregular rhythms and poor heart function. The low-risk group, which makes up 30 percent of the post-heart attack population, has a 2 percent mortality rate in the first year. These patients do not have many extra heartbeats and have good heart function.

Before discharge, many medical centers attach a *Holter monitor,* which is a small recording unit the size of a Walkman, to record the heart activity for twenty-four hours for the purpose of discovering irregular heartbeats, which are then treated. A nuclear scan is also done to test the function of the heart before discharge. Some cardiologists recommend that patients undergo a minimal exercise stress test to discover if angina occurs and if there are major changes on the electrocardiogram, which are a portent of sudden death. If major changes are found, cardiac catheterization is performed. How seriously diseased the arteries are found to be will determine if surgery is necessary. Sometimes the remaining arteries are so critically narrowed (95 percent) that life hangs on a thin thread and arterial replacement is mandatory.

Other cardiologists prefer to do a stress test about three to six weeks after discharge. The damaged heart, they feel, needs a little more time to heal, to form a good scar. Also, they maintain that the function of the heart is likely to improve in the ensuing weeks.

If there is anginal pain after a heart attack, the severity, duration, and the response to nitroglycerine, beta-blockers, and channel calcium blockers will determine if cardiac catheterization should be performed. Some patients may have slight anginal pain, which lasts a minute or two; others, with prolonged chest pain, need to be catheterized and are candidates for surgery.

Recently, numerous studies have given doctors a new tool for the prevention of another attack and sudden death. All the studies using beta-blockers shortly after a heart attack found a 25 to 35 percent reduction in death. I suspect that the use of one-half aspirin per day and the addition of channel calcium blockers will further reduce mortality, providing that the patient: 1. does not have left main artery disease; 2. does not smoke; 3. controls the blood pressure; 4. controls his weight; and 5. takes his medication as prescribed.

Should Routine Cardiac Catheterization Be Performed after a Heart Attack?

Some cardiologists are of the opinion that it is important to know how many arteries are clogged and whether or not new channels should be placed. Others feel cardiac catheterization and bypass surgery should be considered if anginal pain reappears. Others are of the opinion a young person below the age of forty who has sustained a heart attack should have his arteries studied for the purposes of prognosis and should even be considered for bypass surgery if there is serious disease.

I recommend cardiac catheterization after a heart attack if the pre-discharge stress test is very abnormal and the nuclear scan shows a poor heart function. This is the setting for a new heart attack and even sudden death. I also recommend cardiac catheterization be performed if chest pain continues after a heart attack, as pain after a heart attack is an ominous sign of an impending disaster.

There cannot be strict guidelines set when to do catheterization, as each person must be assessed separately. The practice of medicine is a constant balancing of risk versus benefit, and the final decision is based on experience and judgment.

Life after a Heart Attack

Life after a heart attack should be as good or better than before a heart attack. First, of course, dietary control, exercise, the cessation of all smoking, and control of hypertension are mandatory.

Medications will be determined by the physician on an individual basis. If there are no contraindications, beta-blockers are used as described earlier, along with nitroglycerine paste or tablets and calcium channel blockers; also, a half an aspirin per day is helpful in preventing another heart attack and sudden death. Medications are added if there are irregularities of the heart. The patient with a constipation problem needs a stool softener. Forcing at stool can bring on angina and sometimes even another heart attack. There needs to be close cooperation at all times between the doctor and the patient.

Besides the pathological changes that occur in a person's body after a heart attack, there are undoubtedly psychological changes as well. Dealing with the changes become an important part of the rehabilitation program.

The rehabilitation program begins in the coronary care unit with highly specialized nurses' instructing the patient on minor exercises of the legs, arms, and feet, then on sitting up and walking, and lastly, about outside care.

In the coronary care unit, we observe numerous types of behavior. Aggressive individuals sometimes become overbearing and create a hostile atmosphere. The aggressive business tycoon may, on the other hand, become as quiet as a lamb—conservative, understanding, sometimes fearful, grateful for the care he is receiving. Others regard the entire episode as one big joke and jest with everybody in the hospital: "It was senseless to make all this fuss over me. I'm not really sick." Still others may become terrified of the whole scene: tubes, monitors, doctors, nurses. They lie as still as a log, afraid to move, to cough, to talk. Others will flirt with the nurses, be sexually suggestive, and sometimes even display more than emotions.

If the monitoring equipment attached to the body accidentally falls off, it releases a shricking siren that sends a jolt of terror through any sensitive person. Fortunately, the modern coronary care unit no longer inevitably has that insufferable beeping sound constantly in the room. If the beeping sounds are sometimes present, the patient must realize that any movement of his body or a cough can change the beep, and a change should not be interpreted as a sign of imminent cardiac arrest.

The most devastating post-heart-attack response is depression. Depression may manifest itself in the unit or after discharge from the hospital. Now released from the comfortable and secure world of the hospital, the patient is suddenly left floating unattended to cope with his own symptoms in his own fashion. Every time there is a twinge in his chest, the patient thinks another heart attack is imminent. A cramp in the arm, a pain in the jaw, or stomach distress makes the patient think of the possibility of another attack.

Many heart attacks occur at the height of a person's career, so a new perspective on life has to be achieved. Patients must understand after they sustain a heart attack that the aim is to return to their usual activities. Reasons for not returning to the same activity as before may range from severe cardiac impairment to lack of motivation. Some occupations cannot be safely undertaken again. Airplane pilots and others engaged in potentially hazardous work need careful guidance from their physician. The majority of patients want to resume their responsibility as soon as possible. Others may go beyond accepting the disability and may capitalize on the illness. Patients who remain depressed, dependent, and fearful can profit from psychotherapy.

Depressive reactions stem basically from fear of death, which keeps some patients from engaging in some of their favorite activities, in both work and play. The once intrepid individual may feel useless and fearful. Rehabilitation cannot be done alone, but must be undertaken in concert with the family and friends, and if possible with the particular enthusiasm of a parent, spouse, or other person close to the patient. If the partner is fearful, it will be difficult for the recovering patient to shed his or her fears. The partner must be informed about the situation and undergo education similar to the patient's. She or he becomes a participant in the rehabilitation program by attending conferences with the patient and the physician. A too-fearful partner will discourage any activity.

In cases where a married man is the patient, I know some wives who stay up all night to observe if their husbands are still breathing—they become experts on the sleeping habits of their husbands. The wife observes for the first time that sleeping patterns cause respirations to slow down and speed up. Sometimes she becomes more depressed than her husband as she becomes uncertain of her future. Monetary matters enter into the picture, especially if the family's earnings are marginal. Financial burdens may become enormous, and the husband may not be able to return to productive work. By the time compensation and disability payments arrive, there can be great hardship. When the patient does apply for disability, it may take months, involving re-examinations, frustrations, filling out forms—there never seems to be an end.

In the past decades, physicians treating patients with myocardial infarctions felt that physical activity had a deleterious effect on the cardiovascular system. Six to eight weeks of bed rest was the usual prescription. Drs. Sam Levine and K.W.G. Brown, in Boston, in 1929, claimed that too early activity would lead to rupture of the heart, because they reasoned that it takes eight weeks for scar tissue to form. Later, in 1952, Dr. Bernard Lown, also of Boston, and Dr. Levine prescribed the armchair rather than the bed rest treatment for seventy-three patients with heart attacks and found that there were no ill effects in early mobilization. They warned of the hazards of prolonged bed rest, including impaired exercise tolerance, rapid muscle wasting, poor lung perfusion, and clots in the lung.

In-patient rehabiliation programs vary from one center to the other. Each patient must consult his own physician for the program suited for him, which will depend on the total cardiac status. Here is one type of program currently used. This is a guide, not to be used by the patient unless approved by his doctor.

Beginning on day one, there should be active motion of the ankles, anywhere from five to ten times a day; also, the patient should sit in a chair for about fifteen minutes. On the following days, with the help of a physical therapist, additional motions of the shoulders, elbows, and hips are encouraged. Patients are encouraged to flex and extend the feet and knees on an hourly basis. These leg exercises also increase the blood flow through the legs (the use of elastic stockings to prevent clots is also recommended). All this occurs if the patient has an uncomplicated myocardial infarction. The activities are terminated if the pulse rate goes beyond 115 beats per minute. After activities are resumed, each day there is a progression of activity until discharge.

Thousands of patients have had no mishaps with this program. At the same time that the physical exercise is instituted, religious and/or psychological counseling and cardiac instruction programs are started. Diets are explained to the patient, as are medications.

After discharge from the hospital, for the patient who has had an uncomplicated heart attack, the out-patient activity is a continuation of the in-patient program. The patient is encouraged to walk ten minutes in the morning and ten minutes in the afternoon, approximately one-quarter of a mile, and to nap each day for one half hour. During the third week, climbing stairs is permitted, one flight at a time, counting five seconds before each step. Alcoholic beverages are allowed, but a maximum of two to three ounces at dinner. By the third week, the patient should walk thirty minutes in the morning and thirty minutes in the afternoon, approximately one mile. By the fourth week, he should walk forty-five minutes in the morning and forty-five minutes in the afternoon; by the end of the fifth week, one hour in the morning and one hour in the afternoon, with afternoon naps. Usually, at the end of the fifth and sixth weeks, the patient may walk as much as he likes. He is discouraged from walking if the weather is very hot or very cold, and walking should preferably be done early in the morning or late in the afternoon, certainly not directly after meals. If the patient feels fatigued, he should refrain from walking that day. Walking is performed on level ground. The physician will decide the program that is best suited to the patient. This decision may be based on the performance after a stress test.

At the end of a two-month period, a more vigorous exercise program can be instituted. The American Heart Association conducts a program that consists of a minimum of three exercise sessions, each forty-five minutes. Resuscitation equipment, including a portable electrocardiogram machine, defibrillator, and emergency medication kits, is on hand. The forty-five minute sessions are divided in three fifteen-minute periods and consist of calisthenics, walk-jog activity, volleyball, basketball, and swimming. If these are not available, then my own prescription is to start each morning with five arm-raising exercises and walking for five to ten minutes in the morning, resting in the afternoon. Late in the afternoon, five to ten arm-raising exercises and the walking should again be done. In our own laboratory, we conduct exercise stress testing approximately three weeks after the patient has returned from the hospital to determine the exercise prescription. While in the hospital many cardiologists perform a mini-stress test prior to the patient's discharge. This may enable the physician to determine if the patient will need a more aggressive approach to his disease, as angiography or bypass surgery. If the test is markedly positive, the patient has a strong chance of sustaining another attack within the first six months and may be a candidate for bypass surgery.

SEX AFTER A HEART ATTACK

Since our sexual revolution, the discussion of sexual matters can be conducted in an open, sensible fashion. I encourage the wives and husbands of heart attack victims to participate in the physical activities of the rehabilitation program. Sexual intercourse is less demanding on the heart than most people think (especially if you have a regular partner). What's more, physical fitness programs reduce the occurrence of angina, prevent increased heart rates, and make sexual intercourse more enjoyable and safe.

Most patients fear that intercourse will bring on sudden death. The true frequency of sudden death or new heart attack during intercourse is unknown. Energy expended during sexual activity is equal to walking briskly on the street or climbing two flights of stairs. If a patient can perform on an exercise level of six to eight calories per minute, as in vigorous walking or in bicycling, and not exhibit any symptoms—abnormal pulse rate, blood pressure, or electrocardiographic changes—it is safe to recommend to him that he resume his sexual life.

The amount of calories utilized in the pre-orgasmic and post-orgasmic period is approximately 4.5 calories per minute. So, the answer to the patient's question, "When can I engage in sex?" can be summarized, "When you are able to walk briskly on the street or climb one or two flights of stairs." Most of the time, we find that patients can resume full sexual activity at approximately the end of the sixth week.

Some men lose their desire to resume intercourse because of fear of death. I call this the "John Garfield syndrome." Some readers may remember that the actor died during sexual intercourse, and it became a common saying, "If I am going to go, I want to go like Garfield." Other men have personal acquaintances or friends who died suddenly during sexual activity, and this knowledge only adds more to the fear. Still other men take the opposite stance. Their libido is heightened after a heart attack because of the will to "live and be merry"; "life is short, might as well make hay while the sun shines." Against doctor's orders, they resume intercourse too early, and then this can be dangerous.

A certain number of men and women become depressed after a heart attack, and sex is the furthest thing from their minds. The depression can be insidious, starting with a sleep disturbance and extreme exhaustion. Early morning wakening, followed by a lack of interest, inability to concentrate, and even memory loss are signs of depression.

Sexual desire usually returns once the depression subsides. The treatment of depression may require counseling. Once patients are convinced that death is not imminent and return to the mainstream of their lives, their depression often disappears.

In a man, the inability to initiate or maintain an erection may result from medications. Beta-blockers, like *Inderal,* can cause impotence and fatigue. The sexual desire is present, but the medications may prevent a full erection. Sometimes changing the type of beta-blocker can help (for example, Inderal to *Lopressor*).

The wife can play a crucial role to ease the fear of intercourse. She must deal with her own fears, which are quickly felt by the man and which inhibit both partners. Her fears can be allayed if open discussions are held with the couple's physician. More often than not, the wife is too embarrassed to initiate the discussion on sexual matters and receives information indirectly, as from newspaper columns, neighbors, and other sources.

II

PREVENTION AND TREATMENT

4

Coronary Risk Factors

Angina occurs when the arteries become packed with fatty material and the travel of blood-carrying oxygen to the heart is impeded. In addition, as I pointed out earlier, the artery can go into spasm, which can result in further narrowing. The agonizing and frightful pain of angina results from not enough blood being delivered to the heart, which then stimulates nerve endings at different parts of the body—in front of the chest, or in the neck, the shoulder, or the wrists. The purpose of the treatment of angina is to improve the quality of life, to prevent a heart attack, to prolong life, and to avoid bypass surgery.

The treatment of this symptom of coronary artery disease can only be undertaken successfully if the patient understands why the disease started in the first place and what the goals of the physician are. This chapter will discuss the risk factors and what the patient can do about them, focusing principally on stress, cigarette smoking, obesity, cholesterol, and hypertension.

It is imperative that a solid doctor-patient relationship exists. The patient should be confident that the physician knows what he is doing and should be willing to follow his instructions. The more the patient understands the mechanism of his illness, the more likely is the treatment to succeed. A mistrustful or cavalier attitude may result in failure.

Today, the patient can expect most physicians to be competent in the field of cardiology and often will be referred to a cardiologist mainly for extra guidance. A second opinion is a valid option for the patient who is diagnosed to have angina, and when in doubt, the patient should ask for a second opinion from a cardiologist. I have outlined in the previous sections when a stress test, a thallium stress test, and cardiac catheterization should be performed. It would be perfectly in order to ask your physician whether you should have these tests if he fails to suggest them.

Stress

Often, the most effective thing a physician can do is to understand the patient's life style. Recently, a sixty-five-year-old successful insurance agent who was diagnosed as having coronary artery disease, with moderate symptoms aggravated by spasm of the coronary arteries, came to see me. The best treatment was outlined to this man and he understood that even if he underwent bypass surgery and had new vessels placed, those new vessels could also go into spasm and cause the same chest pain as before surgery. He decided to go down the medical path rather than the surgical; yet he did not respond. It became clear, after a careful history-taking, that his episode of angina, or "spasms," as he so well put it, occurred when he arrived at his office in the morning each day between nine and ten o'clock. Once he settled in and the day marched on, his angina subsided. It was during this early hour of the morning that his son-in-law came in to discuss with him various problems which he, the senior agent, felt should have been resolved. His son-in-law clearly did not live up to expectations.

When the insurance agent went on his vacation to

Florida, the chest pain entirely subsided. His relief, he realized, was not related to the southern climate, but to the peace of mind that he was able to find away from his office. Having identified his problem, he did not want to retire, and he certainly could not kick out his son-in-law. An honest conversation among the physician, the son-in-law, and the insurance agent resulted in great improvement. Today this same insurance agent, less critical of and more confident in his son-in-law, has seen his angina virtually disappear.

In a similar story, a fifty-eight-year-old man developed symptoms of coronary artery disease that became most prominent at six o'clock in the evening. The late afternoon tends to be a high-tension time in most of our lives, but it was especially so for this man, for when he arrived home the first words out of his wife's lips inevitably described the difficult day she had suffered with her dreadful arthritic pain. They had been married for twenty-five years, the relationship had begun to sour, and it was now stressful for him to go home. He did not have the courage to leave his wife, for fear of being alone, so he chose to continue in his unhappy way and had become very depressed, which coincided with the development of his symptoms.

Unfortunately—or perhaps fortunately—human beings have an enormous amount of chemical reactions going on in their bodies. Our eyes, our ears, and our senses are continuously responding to outside stimuli either in a negative or positive way. It is part of being alive. That an unpleasant situation creates chemical chaos in our bodies has been known for many years and is now moving to the front line of medical recognition. Different chemicals, like adrenaline, send messages from the brain down to our arteries, sometimes resulting in spasm and chest pain. Adrenaline can make our heart beat fast, our palms sweat, and make us feel fearful and frightened, as if a train was coming toward us. Compulsiveness, strong feelings of inadequacy, frustrations, depressions, trying to complete a job exactly on time—all are detrimental to our entire vascular system. Nervousness causes our hands to get cold. In some, faces become bright red as blood pressure rises, causing the heart to work more than ever. A normal heart can withstand the chronic impact of our modern society, but not one whose arteries are diseased. I do not believe that chronic tension and unhappiness are the cause of coronary artery disease, but I certainly feel they play a major role in perpetuating the symptoms that can lead to a heart attack.

Surely the patient who develops angina should try to change his style of life. I think it is wrong to interfere with the basic personality of an individual who is highly motivated and successful and turn him into a passive person who cares less about what happens to him or the rest of his world; rather the patient needs to learn to balance his chaotic chemistry. Undoubtedly expert counseling from a psychologist can be helpful. The patient, however, can also help himself. For example, instead of beginning the morning in a mad rush, he can arise a half-hour earlier and spend a little extra time at the breakfast table. He can do things in an orderly, calm manner. This hard-driving type of personality is called Type A.

After his bypass surgery, James was advised to change his maddened pace, his need to do three things at one time. A husband or a wife can be a major factor in how well the patient responds to treatment. Understanding, not showing excessive fear, creating an atmosphere of calm and relaxation, planning pleasurable times—these will necessarily improve the patient's condition. The doctor can only advise; it is the patient who has to reset his thermostat.

Fear is the worst enemy in coronary artery disease. The fear of suddenly dying remains constantly in the patient's mind—that slight twinge, that little gas bubble of a pain, brings on the panic that then causes the hormones to be secreted, increasing the heart rate and the pain. The patient has to understand that the heart is an extraordinarily strong organ. The only thing it cannot tolerate is lack of oxygen. Tension, anger, rushing—all decrease the oxygen delivery to the heart. In order to derive the maximum benefit from medication, the inner self has to be mended.

If the patient chooses to undergo bypass surgery, he should know that the anxieties and tensions present prior to surgery are going to be there after surgery. The fast heart-beat, the irregular heartbeats, the arrhythmias, are not going to be improved by bypass surgery or by medications.

THE TYPE A PERSONALITY

A forty-eight-year-old meat cutter had a long family history of heart attacks. The patient's speech was hurried, loud, and explosive, and even as he asked a question he would have another question ready before the first was answered. On the surface, he was a jovial person, but in truth, he despised his job and was frustrated because of economic pressures. He did not respond to medical treatment and chose to have the problem taken care of the "right way." He underwent bypass surgery, which was successful; however, several months later, the pain returned. His life style had not changed, and he was back to where he started.

Patients who try to do what is beyond them must learn to moderate their ambitions and their behavior. One of the major causes of frustration is trying to achieve the impossible. It is as if an average tennis player tried to become a pro. It is important to keep goals in perspective. In the same way, during the rehabilitation program goals should be realistic, not aimed too high. Everyone cannot be a boss, nor should everyone want to be. The inability to ever achieve an unattainable goal is difficult enough for the brain to handle, and it is certainly too difficult to be handled by your coronary arteries without physical penalty.

Dr. Meyer Friedman of Mt. Zion Hospital, San Francisco, and Dr. Ray Rosenman believe that one of the major causes of coronary artery disease is due to emotional reactions. Many physicians feel that stress and meeting deadlines are the major causes of heart attacks, along with other risk factors, such as smoking, high cholesterol, hypertension, a long family history of heart attacks, and inactivity. I believe that if the arteries are normal, Type A behavior is not a risk factor; however, if there is the presence of angina, Type A patients are at greater risk.

In their book, *Type A Behavior and Your Heart*, Drs. Friedman and Rosenman divided behavior into Type A and Type B, Type A characterizing an individual "aggressively involved in the chronic struggle to achieve more in less time." Type B people are more "laid back," perhaps more at peace with the world, not driven to complete a job under a specific deadline, not constantly striving to do everything better.

A Type A male is self-assured, has self-conviction, and yet is insecure. He wants to accomplish a task so that he will be admired, and he always tries to improve. He is aggressive, hostile, competitive, and challenging. He eats rapidly; all his actions are quick. This individual does not allow you to finish a sentence before interrupting. As soon as he asks a question, the next follows. He performs daily tasks simultaneously, such as shaving while having a bowel movement, or speaking on a phone while reading an unrelated document. He cannot tolerate waiting in line. He is basically uncomfortable in his everyday life. Francis Bacon, the great Renaissance philosopher and essayist, advised those who desired a long life to

> . . . avoid anxious fears, angers, sadness . . . [as the] best [state of mind] to preserve health.

Besides behavioral patterns as a cause of coronary artery disease, studies have also cited social factors. One study conducted in North Dakota found coronary heart disease to be higher among men who experience changes in their occupations, lives, or locations. For example, they discovered that men who lived on farms and moved to the city to take office jobs had three times more coronary artery disease. Another study, performed in California, found that Southern rural workers who moved to industrial jobs also developed more coronary artery disease. A study made in the south between 1960 and 1962 recorded twice the prevalence of heart attacks among lower-income people who moved into upper social brackets during that period.

It is all very well to tell a patient, "You must relax. Learn to let things roll off your back," and so on. But how does he learn to change? Fortunately numerous training programs are available that are effective in teaching patients to relax. Here is one I use in my practice:

1. Sit in a chair as comfortably as possible;
2. roll the eyes upward toward the ceiling;
3. slowly close the eyes and take a deep breath;
4. exhale, and concentrate on floating your body;
5. allow the arms to feel light in order to reach a deeper stage.

You can sit like this for several minutes, keeping your body floating, and begin to relax your chin, your neck, your shoulders, your fingertips—right down to the tips of your toes. This should be continued for several minutes and repeated three times a day at a set time. In order to end the session, roll up the eyes again while closed, inhale, open the eyes, exhale, and relax. This is a method used by many psychologists in stress disorder programs that is effective if continued on a regular basis.

Biofeedback, which was first formulated in 1961 by Dr.

Norbert Viener, is a method of training through which a person gains willful control of physiological processes such as blood pressure that are not voluntarily controlled. Electrodes attached to the subject's skin pick up signals from the body which are converted into video signals, such as colored lights, or aural signals, such as beeps or clicks. The patient responds to these images by progressive muscle relaxation and learns to gain control. It is a valuable tool in the treatment of stress. It has been used for the treatment of migraine, tension headaches, hypertension, and so forth. There are biofeedback centers throughout the country.

Cigarette Smoking

As a physician, it is inconceivable to me how, in 1985, a grown mature person who has developed angina can continue smoking. It goes without saying that the person should not have been smoking in the first place. In spite of the propaganda and the skeptics, I do not know of any physician who will differ from the opinion that cigarette smoking is enormously harmful to the heart and to the lungs. The mechanism of how cigarette smoking increases the severity of hardening of the arteries is not fully known. It is known that cigarettes themselves can cause spasm of the coronary arteries and bring on angina. Scientists have shown that carbon monoxide from the cigarette is an important cause of the detrimental changes in the metabolism of the arterial wall. In my own practice, I have not seen any patient's heart improve while he is still smoking. Smoking accelerates the progression of coronary artery disease and is a very important reason why people develop heart attacks. It stands to reason that if the lungs are filled with smoke not enough oxygen gets to the important places—to the arteries, to the brain, and to the kidneys. Once you have been diagnosed as having coronary artery disease, the best way to end up on the operating table is to continue smoking cigarettes.

Cigarette smoking increases the heart rate. As the heart rate increases, the heart needs more oxygen. If the arteries are narrowed by atherosclerosis, angina results. Furthermore, smoking interferes with the efficacy of the medications given for the treatment of angina. To prove this point, some heart doctors in the cardiology department at the Hammersmith Hospital in London conducted an experiment in which patients smoked while taking their medication. A stress test was performed, as were other cardiac function tests. It was discovered that smoking actually reduced the level of medicines in the blood and that the angina continued. (This excellent study was reported in the *New England Journal of Medicine* of April 12, 1984.)

Smoking also makes the cells of the blood stick against the walls of the arteries, thus further decreasing the flow of blood. Smoking cigarettes is a prevalent, terrifying, and disabling illness, from my point of view, and yet it is very difficult to be able to convince smokers to quit this dangerous and disgusting habit. On the one hand, the government tells us not to smoke; on the other, it supports the tobacco-growing industry. This certainly does not help matters at all!

There are numerous techniques described to help the patient give up smoking, like Smoke-Enders and hypnosis, which all are helpful. I know only one action that really works, however, and that is for smokers to throw away their cigarettes—right now—and then encourage others to join the cause for cleaner air, cleaner lungs, and better hearts. Eliminate the cigarettes and angina will improve, and we will be on the way to bypassing bypass surgery.

A WORD ABOUT WOMEN

American women in the past twenty-five years have increased their rate of heart attacks as their roles in business and the professions have increased. (A survey of Japanese women who are now engaged in business activities revealed that they have increased their incidence of heart disease fourfold.) But although heart attacks in women over the age of fifty are increasingly being reported, they are relatively rare in women under the age of fifty.

In a study performed by the public health department of Boston University School of Medicine, it was concluded that in young women, "cigarette smoking is the dominant risk factor." Eighty-four percent who suffered heart attacks were smokers. The other risk factors included the total cholesterol, the HDL levels, the hypertension. Women who had a family history of heart attack or stroke before the age of sixty were found to be susceptible. The hyperactive Type A personality was not associated with heart attacks in women, and obesity was not associated with a significant percentage. Rare cases of women taking oral contraceptive pills having heart attacks have been reported. It would appear from this study that in order for women to avoid coronary bypass surgery, the first step is to stop smoking.

Overweight and Obesity

The successful medical treatment of angina requires the patient to achieve an ideal weight. Obesity and overweight are major risk factors in the development of angina. Overweight patients often have higher cholesterol levels and a tendency to develop hypertension.

A grossly overweight man, a nonsmoker, successful in business, developed angina at the age of fifty-eight. He was 5′7″ and weighed 260 pounds. His blood pressure was elevated. The patient did not lose weight, and his angina progressed to a heart attack. After his heart attack, all his risk factors continued, his angina returned, and a bypass operation was performed. Several months after the bypass surgery, he remained obese. His new blood vessels were visualized again through re-catheterization and were found to be blocked. The patient was advised to have another operation. When he consulted me, he had evidence of angina, and it was apparent that the medications were not helping him. After being overweight for nearly thirty years, he embarked on a very strict weight reduction program. His diet eliminated all fats, sweets, and salt. This man took a most heroic stand, and with great persistence achieved a much more acceptable life. You can never be too thin if you are suffering from angina.

There are no magical diets to weight reduction. It all has to do with caloric restrictions. The elements that contribute to weight loss are water, fat, protein, and glycogen, a sugar protein. In the early phases of caloric restriction, the initial loss of weight may vary to a marked degree. As you continue your diet, water may be retained and you may actually gain some weight initially, although there is a net loss of fat and protein. Subjects placed on a weight-reduction program often rapidly lose weight during the first week or two, and then the weight tends to stay at a plateau for a few weeks. This initial weight reduction is due to salt and water losses.

It is customary to assume that, on the average, one pound, or 0.45 kilos, of weight loss corresponds to an energy loss of approximately 3,500 calories. This means that 90 percent of the calories burned are derived from the fat deposits in the body. In order to lose one pound, there has to be a deficiency of 3,500 calories. An average person uses approximately 2,500 calories per day; if you ingest 4,000 calories, which is 1,500 calories in excess, you cannot possibly lose weight. On the other hand, if the caloric intake is limited to 1,000 calories, and you utilize 2,000 calories, weight loss is inevitable. For example, if you limit your daily intake to 1,000 calories and burn up 2,000 calories in daily activities, there will be a total deficit of 1,000 calories and there will be a weight loss of one-third pound per day. A caloric counter is a simple way of estimating the total calories ingested.

As the diet is continued, fat is utilized and protein is preserved, which is the most important beneficial effect of strict caloric control. Rather than relying on dietary fads and natural-food gimmicks, the simplest way to lose weight is to count calories. Weight reduction should be done gradually, over an extended period of time, because it takes many years to become overweight in the first place. The diet has to be sensibly balanced with sufficient proteins, carbohydrates, fats, and vegetables; but restrict calories!

Fad diets can be dangerous and should be avoided. Weight reduction requires a re-education and elimination of bad eating habits. For example, not eating all day and then eating 2,000 calories at night is foolish. It is better to divide the total calories between several meals.

The role of exercise will be discussed later on. Suffice it to say now that exercise with no dietary restriction will not cause appreciable weight loss. I have seen numerous overweight tennis players.

The Cholesterol Story

Cholesterol and arteriosclerosis are related. Arteriosclerosis is a major disease, affecting not only the coronary arteries but also the entire arterial system in the adult, beginning in childhood. The earliest atherosclerosis found in the arteries consists of fatty streaks, which are then followed by a fibrous plaque (a hardened mass) which becomes more advanced; the fibrous plaque is composed mostly of lipids, collagen fibers, and other cells.

It is this plaque that occludes the arterial lumen (channels). The role of cholesterol as the cause of arteriosclerosis has now been well confirmed by epidemiological and biochemical studies. Why the ingested fat accumulates in the artery is still not known.

It has taken decades before physicians have finally accepted the fact that excessive cholesterol and saturated fat intake is harmful to the body. Some persons are more susceptible to the ingestion of cholesterol than others. A person who has established angina undoubtedly is one of the people susceptible to the ingestion of cholesterol. Most of the cholesterol found in the body is produced in the liver, while 30 percent generally comes from the food that we eat. I have heard patients and acquaintances say, "My doctor does not believe in the cholesterol theory." That was all very well until current knowledge conclusively proved that high cholesterol does cause atherosclerosis! Bear in mind that although treatment of angina may be successful in terms of medications that eliminate symptoms of the illness, the medications will not eliminate the progression of atherosclerosis.

American soldiers killed during the Korean War and the Vietnam War were found to have the beginning of plaques in their arteries at nineteen and twenty, while Korean and Vietnamese young men did not. Similarly, the populations of Asia, Africa, and Latin America live mostly on vegetables and starch grain products, and their intake of fat is very low. Arteriosclerosis and coronary artery disease is rare in these countries. The average cholesterol found in the blood of these people is in the range of 140 to 160 mg, as compared to 250 mg and above in Americans. We have known for many years that the Japanese, who have a national diet low in fat, had the lowest rate of cardiovascular disease; however, when the Japanese immigrated to the United States and began to eat our Western diet, their incidence of heart disease increased to ten times that of their former countrymen in Japan.

The cholesterol story is an old story. It was known as

early as 1930, when the Russian pathologist Dr. Nikolai Anitschkow showed that he could produce human-like deposits of plaques in the arteries of rabbits by feeding them a diet rich in cholesterol. The story is told that the Czar of Russia once complained that members of his elite guard were dying prematurely, while the peasants lived to old age —the peasants, of course, subsisted on grains and vegetables, while the elite guard were treated with rich meats and caviar.

It is now nearly a quarter of a century since Dr. Paul Dudley White and other researchers argued that high cholesterol needed to be controlled in order to prevent an epidemic of premature arteriosclerosis and heart disease.

Dr. Ancel Keyes, who was an epidemiologist, conducted a relevant study in seven nations in 1947. He, too, discovered a direct correlation among the incidence of heart disease, the level of cholesterol, and the amount of animal fat ingested. The highest rate of heart disease was discovered to be in Finland. The Finns eat more fat than any other European nation. Sandwiches of pure fat for lunch are common.

In the United States, deaths from coronary artery disease began to rise sharply in the early 1940s, reaching a peak in 1968, and then, for some reason yet unknown, began to decline, until the number is now 25 percent lower than it was in 1968. The decline in death rate seems to coincide with a drop in the cholesterol levels of middle-aged American males, who also, as a group, cut back on cigarette smoking, more strictly controlled their blood pressure, and exercised more.

For twenty-five years, the controversy has raged about whether cholesterol in our diet is responsible for arteriosclerosis. The National Heart, Lung and Blood Institute, a part of the National Institutes of Health (NIH), conducted a ten-year investigation (the Lipid Research Clinic's Coronary Primary Prevention Trial) of 3,806 men between the ages of 35 and 59, all of whom had cholesterol levels above 265 mg. These men were divided into two groups, one-half receiving daily doses of a medication that lowers the cholesterol, called *cholestyramine*, and the other group no treatment. At the end of this study, the drug-treated group had their cholesterol lowered by 8.5 percent.

The cardiologist who directed this study, Dr. Robert Levy, concluded, "If we can get everyone to lower their cholesterol by 10 to 15 percent by cutting down on fat and cholesterol in their diet, heart attack deaths in this country will decrease by 30 percent." In fact, in 1984, the study unequivocally demonstrated that lowering the cholesterol level will lower the risk of heart attack by 35 percent.

Scientists recognize there are different types of cholesterol:

1. HDL—high-density lipoprotein, which is the good kind. It eliminates the bad cholesterol from the circulation. The higher the HDL function recorded, the lower the risk of a heart attack. Exercise and several ounces of alcohol per day raise the level of HDL. Smoking lowers the level of HDL.

2. LDL—low-density lipoprotein, which is dangerous to your health. The higher the LDL, the more risk of heart disease. The LDL is the delivery truck that carries the cholesterol and deposits it on the arteries.

At the time of birth, everybody has low levels of cholesterol (including the culprit, LDL), but as adulthood is reached, cholesterol levels increase. Males and females at the time of birth have the same level of fat in their blood, but as the boys reach maturity, there is a drop of 25 percent in the good cholesterol in men and a rise of the LDL. Some researchers postulate that this is the reason there are fewer coronary deaths in women than in men.

Approximately 2 percent of Americans may have genetic protection against developing arteriosclerosis. All of us have known people who have lived to a ripe old age despite habitually eating eggs and bacon and smoking.

Not only is a low-fat diet essential for the prevention of coronary artery disease, it is mandatory for the treatment of coronary artery disease and avoiding bypass surgery. Below is a table compiled by the United States Department of Agriculture on the amount of cholesterol in different foods that we daily eat. It can be readily seen that it is quite easy to ingest more than 300 mg of cholesterol per day.

Table 1. Cholesterol content of common foods

Food	*Amount*	*Cholesterol (in milligrams)*
	Meat Group	
	Red Meats	
Bacon	2 slices	15
Beef (lean)	3 ounces	77
Frankfurter	2 (4 ounces)	112
Ham, boiled	2 ounces	51
Kidney, beef	3 ounces	315
Lamb (lean)	3 ounces	85
Liver, beef	3 ounces	372
Pork (lean)	3 ounces	75
Veal (lean)	3 ounces	84
	Fowl	
Chicken (dark meat, no skin)	3 ounces	77
Chicken (light meat, no skin)	3 ounces	65
Eggs (whole or yolk only)	1 large	252
Turkey (dark meat, no skin)	3 ounces	86
Turkey (white meat, no skin)	3 ounces	65

Food	*Amount*	*Cholesterol (in milligrams)*
	Fish	
Clams, raw	3 ounces	43
Crab, canned	3 ounces	85
Flounder	3 ounces	69
Haddock	3 ounces	42
Halibut	3 ounces	50
Lobster	3 ounces	71
Mackerel	3 ounces	84
Oysters, raw	3 ounces	42
Salmon, canned	3 ounces	30
Sardines	3 ounces	119
Scallops	3 ounces	45
Shrimp, canned	3 ounces	128
Tuna, canned	3 ounces	55
	Milk Group	
Butter	1 tablespoon	35
Buttermilk	1 cup	5
Cheese, cottage (4% fat)	1/2 cup	24
Cheese, cottage (1% fat)	1/2 cup	12
Cheese, cream	1 ounce	31
Cheese, hard	1 ounce	24–28
Cheese, spread	1 ounce	18
Chocolate milk (low-fat)	1 cup	20
Cream, heavy	1 tablespoon	21
Ice cream	1/2 cup	27
Ice milk	1/2 cup	13
Milk, skim	1 cup	5
Milk (1% fat)	1 cup	14
Milk (2% fat)	1 cup	22
Milk, whole	1 cup	34
Yogurt (low-fat)	1 cup	17
	Bread Group	
Angel food cake	1 slice	0
Chocolate cupcake	2 1/2-inch diameter	17
Cornbread	1 ounce	58

Food	*Amount*	*Cholesterol (in milligrams)*
	Bread Group (cont)	
Lemon meringue pie	1/8 of 9-inch pie	98
Muffin, plain	3-inch diameter	21
Noodles, egg	1 cup	50
Pancakes	7 tablespoons batter	54
Sponge cake	1/12 of 10-inch cake	162

The National Heart, Lung and Blood Institute study clearly tells us that arteriosclerosis can be halted *and reversed.* As long as ten years ago, it was shown that the fatty deposits in the coronary arteries of monkeys shrank when the animals were placed on a drastic cholesterol-lowering diet, and there are cases reporting shrinkage of cholesterol deposits in arteries of humans. Arteriosclerosis of the coronary arteries is therefore a preventable disease.

Again, moderate exercise raises the HDL (the good cholesterol) as does two to three ounces of alcohol (one or two cocktails) per day. Stress plays a factor in lowering the HDL: it has been shown that the cholesterol levels of medical students get higher right before the exams, as do accountants' as the April 15 deadline nears.

The American Heart Association has recommended that people have a daily intake of not more than 300 mg of cholesterol, which is about equal to one egg, but the average American diet consists of 450 mg or more. I believe a much more drastic reduction in the cholesterol intake is needed if we are going to eliminate angina and the need for bypass surgery. The average American cholesterol level is approximately 230 mg; we should aim for approximately 170, or even 150. The NIH study tells us that for every 1 percent reduction in the total cholesterol level, there is a 2 percent reduction in heart disease risk. The total fat intake should not be more than 30 percent of the diet. Americans are beginning to heed this advice—the national consumption of butter has dropped 30 percent, egg consumption has declined 14 percent. And, as mentioned before, the death rate from heart disease has declined by 25 to 30 percent in the last ten years as Americans have become more conscious of their diets.

Lowering the cholesterol intake to 170 mg is not such a difficult task, and one can still enjoy a gourmet diet. Some basic rules will be helpful to the reader. When going to a restaurant, one should avoid red meats and veal; stick to chicken or fish. A good rule is that you can eat anything that swims, including shellfish. Salmon and mackerel contain fatty acids that reduce cholesterol. Foods can be deceiving; for example, innocent-looking pastas are stuffed with whole-milk cheeses, fatty meats, oily sauces, and cured bacon. Antipasto can be eaten, provided it does not have anchovies. Choose pastas that have marinara sauce, red or white clam or mussel sauce. Keep in mind that very many desserts contain eggs, cream, and butter. True water ices are ideal, but not milk-based sherbets. French restaurants are notorious for using large amounts of butter and cream. Good choices of French hors d'oeuvres include mussels that are grilled or steamed, and vegetables. Chinese restaurants can be even more deceiving. Steamed fish and chicken dishes may contain eggs; also, eggs frequently turn up in fried rice and noodles. Mexican food often uses pure lard. Safe dishes would include avocado purees and all the hot and mild relish sauces.

Indian restaurants have ghee, which is butter used in the curry sauces and bread. Stick to the roasted seafood and chicken. The Japanese cuisine has the largest medically desirable choice because of their raw fish creations. But all in all, unless one is selective, switching to an Eastern diet can be just as hazardous as sticking to our American cuisine.

The fish oils contained in salmon or lox seem to have beneficial effects in lowering the LDL, and recently olive oil has been reported to be very beneficial for lowering cholesterol and raising the HDL. Fiber in the diet can reduce the LDL by 20 percent in patients who consume a cup of oat bran a day, according to Dr. John Story of Purdue University.

In persons suffering from angina who have cholesterol counts above 220 mg, strict dietary control is recommended. Since the National Heart, Lung and Blood Institute study has reported its finding that cholesterol is the villain in arteriosclerosis, I also favor the addition of cholestyramine, which is a natural bile found in our bodies, to help lower an elevated cholesterol. If mixed with orange juice, it is palatable. Starting with a low dose and gradually increasing the amount lessens its unpleasantness. Side effects such as constipation and bloating do sometimes occur, as do nausea and gas. The other medications used to lower cholesterol have much more serious side effects, some associated with development of stones in the gallbladder, and with cancer, too. Recently niacin (nicotinic acid) has been reported to be effective in lowering cholesterol and triglycerides. It has the unpleasant side effect of causing flushing of the face and body in some persons; otherwise, it is a safe and effective way to lower cholesterol in the blood. Patients who have undergone bypass surgery also need to be placed on a strict cholesterol-reducing diet, because bypass surgery does not prevent the progression of this illness. Without a change in diet, the remaining arteries that have not been grafted will show signs of progression of arteriosclerosis in 35 percent of patients!

Because arteriosclerosis is closely linked to a high cholesterol level, patients should be screened to determine the level of their serum cholesterol, triglycerides, high-density lipoprotein, and low-density lipoprotein. These measurements are done after a twelve- to fourteen-hour fast, preferably with the last meal prior to the test low in fat. Seventy-five percent of the total cholesterol measured is carried as the

LDL. The total cholesterol, therefore, is a reflection of the low-density lipoprotein.

Effects of Drugs on Blood Lipids

CHOLESTRYAMINE AND COLESTIPOL
Lowers plasma LDL cholesterol by 20 to 25 percent
Causes slight HDL cholesterol rise
May elevate plasma triglyceride levels

NICOTINIC ACID, NIACIN
Lowers LDL cholesterol by about 20 percent
Raises HDL cholesterol by about 30 percent
Lowers plasma triglyceride and VLDL levels by 40 percent

CLOFIBRATE
Lowers plasma triglycerides
Lowers VLDL cholesterol
Little effect on plasma cholesterol or LDL cholesterol
Causes modest HDL elevation

GEMFIBROZIL (LOPID)
Little effect on LDL
Lowers VLDL
Increases HDL considerably

PROBUCOL
Decreases LDL by 15 to 20 percent
May significantly reduce HDL
Little effect on VLDL

The high-density lipoprotein accounts for 20 to 25 percent of the total cholesterol. The higher this figure, the lower is the incidence of coronary artery disease; for example, at levels of 30 mg of the HDL level, the incidence is almost doubled. Therefore, all cholesterol measurements should include an LDL and an HDL.

In summary: a strict low-fat diet lowers the cholesterol, exercise and two to four ounces of alcohol raise the HDL. Cigarette smoking and obesity lower the HDL.

Hypertension

Hypertension (high blood pressure) is one of the identifiable risk factors for the likelihood of developing premature coronary artery disease in both men and women, along with other factors we have noted, such as high serum cholesterol, physical inactivity, obesity, cigarette-smoking, and diabetes. The incidence of heart attacks rises as the level of systolic and diastolic pressure rises. There are approximately sixty million Americans suffering from hypertension; many are not aware of their ailment.

In 1930, Dr. Samuel Levine, the renowned cardiologist from Boston, was the first to note that hypertension is related to heart attacks. His study concluded that more than 60 percent of his 145 heart attack patients were suffering from hypertension. Hypertension undoubtedly accelerates atherosclerosis. Coronary atherosclerosis occurs at least twice as often in patients who have hypertension.

The first physiologist to conduct the most important work on hypertension was Dr. Stephen Hales (1677–1761). He was an English clergyman who originated artificial respiration and made other discoveries. His work on the mechanics of blood pressure marks a milestone in the advancement of the understanding of circulation. By placing a long glass tube in the artery of a horse's leg and observing that the blood rose in the glass tube, he devised the first instrument to measure the blood pressure.

What is blood pressure? Pressure is force per area. The smaller the area, the higher the pressure. Pressure is generated as the result of the pumping action of the heart, which drives the blood to all parts of the body through fifty million arteries, one million capillaries, and 95,000 veins. The entire circulatory system has been calculated to be approximately 150,000 miles in length. As the blood is driven forward from the contracting heart, the blood vessels expand and stretch like a rubber band. As the artery recoils, the blood is further propelled down the stream. Each time the heart contracts, two ounces of blood are sent forward to the arterial system. The arterioles, the terminal ends of the arteries, contract and expand to control the flow of blood.

Two numbers are used for blood pressure readings: the upper level (the systolic reading) and the lower level (the diastolic reading). The force of blood leaving the heart is called the systolic blood pressure. It is the force that is generated by the contraction of the heart by the forward push. The diastolic figure refers to the resistance of flow through the small blood vessels. If the arterioles exert a substantial degree of resistance, the pressure will be high. Both systolic and diastolic pressures are important. The blood pressure varies from minute to minute. Among other things, it is influenced by sitting, standing, eating, lying down, heat, cold, hunger, laughter, happiness, and grief. The blood pressure is recorded at the lowest level between 3:00 and 4:00 A.M. and tends to rise to a peak between 6:00 and 7:00 P.M.

Some patients may record hypertension only at 10:00 A.M., others at noon. Twenty-four-hour blood pressure readings are important to determine the individual person's blood pressure variations. These readings can help to establish a solid treatment program.

Maintaining a normal or slightly lowered blood pressure is a sign of good health. A normal blood pressure reading would be below 140/90. Borderline or mild hypertension is considered at systolic levels of 145 to 160 and diastolic levels of 95 to 100.

The blood pressure is measured by an apparatus called a *sphygmomanometer*. Anyone can learn to take his own blood pressure. Instructions can be given by a nurse or a doctor. The blood pressure cuff around the arm is pumped up until the artery is blocked. As the pressure is slowly released, the thumping sound of the returning blood is heard through the stethoscope. The first thumping sound refers to the systolic blood pressure. It is the amount of pressure that is needed to raise the mercury in the sphygmomanometer. When the contraction of the heart is over and it rests, the pressure is slowly released, and the last sound is called the diastolic pressure, corresponding to the relaxation of the heart.

Home blood-pressure readings are useful, providing the persons themselves understand that blood pressure may vary hourly, daily. It is the consistent elevation that is important, not the occasional one. Physicians should take the blood pressure three or four times during an office visit. Routinely, patients upset when they first come to a physician's office will be further disturbed to find their blood pressure is elevated. The physician must tell the patient this is a very common initial finding, and after retaking the blood pressure several times, a proper assessment can be made. Blood pressure should be examined when the patient is both sitting and standing.

The proper control of hypertension requires weight reduction and salt restriction. The physician then may choose to add a diuretic or to begin any one of a variety of drugs. Regardless of the form of treatment the physician uses, the aim is the same—to control hypertension. Patients who are suffering from angina and hypertension will have their angina markedly relieved when the blood pressure is controlled. It is fortunate that today beta-blockers serve to control both angina and hypertension. Strokes have been decreased by 40 percent because of an extensive nationwide program of controlling hypertension.

The myth that an elevated blood pressure is important in older patients in order to maintain the circulation of the brain is just that, a myth. In older people systolic pressure elevation is a very important predictor of future disease of the coronary arteries and of the brain.

The combination of a cholesterol of 190, a blood pressure of 120, exercise, and a cigarette-free life makes a person less than a 2.5 percent risk in terms of developing a heart attack in eight years, while a patient who has a cholesterol of over 300, a blood pressure of over 180, who doesn't exercise, and who smokes has a 60 percent chance of getting a heart attack within eight years.

Elevation of the blood pressure that is sustained or poorly controlled contributes to enlargement of the heart, arteriosclerosis, and eventual heart failure. One of the most common causes of heart failure still remains high blood pressure. Hypertension causes the muscles of the heart to thicken, the chambers to widen, and the heart to contract inefficiently. Some of these changes can be reversed by adequate control of hypertension.

FORMS OF TREATMENT

Every effort is made to treat hypertension without the use of medications. A vigorous program of weight control is the first step. In one survey it was estimated that 50 percent of hypertension in this country could be eliminated if people lost weight. It is not really known why overweight persons develop hypertension.

Doctors have concluded that 75 percent of patients suffering from mild to moderate hypertension can achieve normal blood pressure readings by weight reduction alone. The question facing physicians is: Who should be treated for hypertension? The answer is that even patients who have mild hypertension (about 150 systolic/95 diastolic) should be started on a program of preventive blood-pressure maintenance, starting with weight control and a low-salt diet.

We are a salty society—saltaholics. The average adult eats two and a half teaspoons (5000 to 6000 mg) of salt per day, which is *twenty times* more than our body needs. Salt is to hypertension what cholesterol is to heart disease—and both are preventable illnesses in most patients.

In 1972, Dr. John Farquhar of Stanford University conducted a three-year study in two towns. In patients who cut their salt intake by 30 percent, the blood pressure was lowered by 6.4 percent. Why salt contributes to hypertension scientists have not yet discovered. It is estimated that 20 to 40 percent of the population is susceptible to the deleterious effects of salt. Blacks are two times more prone to develop hypertension than whites.

Salt restriction coupled with weight loss is essential for the simple treatment of hypertension. A low-salt intake, consisting of 2 gm per day (2000 mg), is necessary. In mild hypertension, a trial of six weeks of weight reduction and salt restriction should be made before other medications are added.

Below is a list of foods and the amount of salt that they contain. One glance will tell the reader that it is no surprise that hypertension is so prevalent in our Western society.

Table 2. Salt (and calorie) content of common foods. Reprinted from the *Journal of the American Medical Association* (248, no. 5), 6 Aug. 1982.

Sodium (and Calorie) Content of Common Foods*

Food item	*Common Measure (Weight, g)*	*Sodium, mg*	*Calories*
	Beverages (Alcoholic)		
Beer, regular	12-oz can or bottle (360)	18	151†
Beer, light	12-oz can or bottle (360)	14	70–136†
Brandy	1 1/2 fl oz (45)	1	105
Gin (86 proof)	1 1/2 fl oz (45)	1	105
Rum (86 proof)	1 1/2 fl oz (45)	1	105
Vodka (86 proof)	1 1/2 fl oz (45)	Trace	105
Whiskey, bourbon, rye, or scotch (86 proof)	1 1/2 fl oz (45)	1	105
Wine, red domestic	4 fl oz (120)	12	99
Wine, red imported	4 fl oz (120)	6	99
Wine, sherry	4 fl oz (120)	14	161
Wine, white domestic	4 fl oz (120)	19	99
Wine, white imported	4 fl oz (120)	2	99

Food item	*Common Measure (Weight, g)*	*Sodium, mg*	*Calories*
	Beverages (Nonalcoholic)		
Apple juice	6 fl oz (180)	4	87
Coffee, brewed	1 cup—8 fl oz (240)	2	0
Coffee, instant	1 cup—8 fl oz (240)	1	2
Cranberry juice cocktail	6 fl oz (180)	3	123
Grape juice, bottled or canned	6 fl oz (190)	6	125
Orange juice, fresh	6 fl oz (180)	4	84
Orange juice, frozen	6 fl oz (186)	4	92
Pineapple juice	6 fl oz (188)	3	69
Prune juice	6 fl oz (192)	4	149
Soft drink‡			
Regular	8 fl oz (240)	11	96
Diet	8 fl oz (240)	29	1
Club soda	8 fl oz (240)	56	0
Collins mix	8 fl oz (240)	20	112
Quinine water (tonic)	8 fl oz (240)	2	72
Mineral water	8 fl oz (240)	42	0
Tomato juice	6 fl oz (192)	659	36
Tea	1 cup—8 fl oz (240)	1	0
Tea, instant	1 cup—8 fl oz (240)	2	0
Vegetable juice cocktail	6 fl oz (182)	665	30
	Breads and Crackers		
Biscuit, home recipe	1 biscuit (28)	175	103
Biscuit, mix, with milk	1 biscuit (28)	272	104
Bread, French	1 slice (23)	116	64
Bread, pumpernickel	1 slice (32)	182	79
Bread, rye	1 slice (25)	139	61
Bread, white	1 slice (25)	114	76
Bread, whole wheat	1 slice (25)	132	61
Bread stick, salt coating	1 stick, small (10)	167	38
Bread stick, without salt coating	1 stick, small (10)	70	38
Cracker, saltine or soda	1 cracker (3)	35	12
Cracker, soup or oyster	10 crackers (8)	83	33
Roll, dinner, brown and serve	1 roll (28)	138	83
Roll, frankfurter, hamburger	1 roll (40)	202	119
Roll, hard	1 roll (50)	313	156

Food item	*Common Measure (Weight, g)*	*Sodium, mg*	*Calories*
	Cereals (Non-Sugar Coated) §		
Bran, all	1 oz—1/3 cup (28)	160	70
Bran flakes (40%)	1 oz—2/3 cup (28)	265	90
Corn flakes	1 oz—1 cup (28)	350	110
Corn Chex	1 oz—1 cup (28)	325	110
Granola	1 oz—1/4 cup (28)	75	130
Grits, cooked	1 oz—3/4 cup (28)	10	100
Oat flakes	1 oz—2/3 cup (28)	275	100
Oatmeal, regular, without salt	1 oz—1/3 cup (28)	1	109
Oatmeal, instant, regular flavor (salt added)	1 oz—3/4 cup (28)	252	105
Rice, cream of, unsalted	1 oz—3/4 cup (28)	10	110
Rice, puffed	1/2 oz—1 heaping cup (14)	10	50
Rice Chex	1 oz—1 1/8 cup (28)	275	110
Rice Crispies	1 oz—1 cup (28)	340	110
Wheat Chex	1 oz—2/3 cup (28)	240	110
Wheat, cream of, regular	1 oz—3/4 cup (28)	7	110
Wheat flakes	1 oz—1 cup (28)	370	110
Wheat, puffed	1/2 oz—1 heaping cup (14)	10	50
Wheat, shredded	1 large biscuit (21)	1	80
	Condiments, Dressings, and Seasonings		
Barbeque sauce	1 tbsp (16)	130	14
Catsup, tomato	1 tbsp (15)	156	16
Chili sauce	1 tbsp (17)	227	16
Mayonnaise	1 tbsp (15)	78	101
Mustard, prepared	1 tsp (5)	65	5
Parsley flakes	1 tbsp (4)	2	2
Pepper, black	1 tsp (2)	1	8
Salad dressings			
Bleu cheese or Roquefort	1 tbsp (15)	153	76
French	1 tbsp (14)	214	66
Italian	1 tbsp (15)	116	83
Russian	1 tbsp (15)	133	74
Thousand Island	1 tbsp (16)	109	80
Oil and vinegar	1 tbsp (15)	Trace	62
Salt, table	1 tsp (6)	2,325	0

Food item	*Common Measure (Weight, g)*	*Sodium, mg*	*Calories*
	Condiments, Dressings, and Seasonings (cont)		
Soy sauce	1 tbsp (18)	1,029	12
Sugar, granulated	1 tsp (4)	Trace	15
Worcestershire sauce	1 tbsp (17)	206	Trace
	Dairy Products, Eggs,‖ and Margarine¶		
Butter, regular	1 tbsp (14)	116	102
Butter, whipped	1 tbsp (9)	74	69
Butter, unsalted, regular	1 tbsp (14)	2	102
Cheese, American	1 slice—1 oz (28)	406	116
Cheese, cheddar	1 oz (28)	176	114
Cheese, cottage	1/2 cup (113)	457	117
Cheese, cream	1 oz (28)	84	99
Cheese, parmesan, grated	1 oz (28)	528	129
Cheese, Swiss	1 oz (28)	74	107
Cheese, processed spread	1 oz (28)	381	82
Cream, half and half	1 tbsp (15)	7	20
Cream, heavy	1 tbsp (15)	6	53
Cream, sour	1 tbsp (12)	6	26
Egg, whole	1 medium (50)	69	79
Egg, white	1 medium (33)	50	16
Egg, yolk	1 medium (17)	8	63
Margarine, regular	1 tbsp (14)	133	100
Margarine, soft, tub	1 tbsp (14)	152	100
Margarine, unsalted	1 tbsp (14)	1	100
Milk, buttermilk	8 fl oz (245)	257	99
Milk, low-fat (2%)	8 fl oz (244)	122	121
Milk, skim	8 fl oz (245)	126	86
Milk, whole	8 fl oz (244)	120	150
	Desserts #		
Brownies	1 average (20)	50	97
Cake, angel food	1 slice, 1/12 cake (56)	134	150
Cake, devil's food, chocolate icing	1 slice, 1/12 cake (67)	120	260
Cake, pound	1 medium slice (55)	171	225
Cake, white, white icing	1 slice, 1/12 cake (104)	243	290
Cake, yellow, with caramel icing	1 slice, 1/12 cake (108)	79	391
Cookies, chocolate chip	1 cookie, medium (11)	35	50

Food item	*Common Measure (Weight, g)*	*Sodium, mg*	*Calories*
	Desserts # (cont)		
Cookies, sandwich	1 cookie (10)	40	63
Cookies, oatmeal	1 cookie (13)	27	120
Cookies, sugar	1 cookie (26)	108	128
Cookies, fig	1 bar (14)	48	56
Cookies, vanilla wafer	1 wafer (4)	9	16
Cookies, shortbread	1 cookie (8)	29	37
Gelatin, plain	1/2 cup (120)	60**	80
Ice cream	1 cup (140)	112	257
Ice milk	1 cup (131)	105	199
Pie, apple	1 slice, 1/8 pie (71)	208	182
Pie, banana cream	1 slice, 1/6 pie (66)	90	128
Pie, blueberry	1 slice, 1/8 pie (71)	163	172
Pie, cherry	1 slice, 1/8 pie (71)	169	185
Pie, chocolate cream	1 slice, 1/6 pie (66)	80	174
Pie, lemon meringue	1 slice, 1/8 pie (105)	296	268
Pie, mince	1 slice, 1/8 pie (71)	241	259
Pie, peach	1 slice, 1/8 pie (71)	169	150
Pie, pecan	1 slice, 1/8 pie (71)	241	259
Pie, pumpkin	1 slice, 1/8 pie (71)	169	150
Pudding, bread	1/2 cup (133)	267	248
Pudding, chocolate, home recipe	1/2 cup (130)	73	198
Pudding, chocolate, mix	1/2 cup (148)	195	322
Pudding, rice	1/2 cup (132)	94	194
Pudding, tapioca	1/2 cup (83)	129	111
Pudding, vanilla, home recipe	1/2 cup (128)	83	142
Pudding, vanilla, mix	1/2 cup (148)	200	321
Sherbet, orange	1 cup (193)	89	259
	Fish and Seafood		
Bluefish, broiled or baked with butter	4 oz (114)	117	219
Clams, raw	4 to 5—3 oz (85)	174	56
Cod, broiled with butter	4 oz (114)	125	99
Crabmeat, canned, drained	1 can—4 oz (114)	1,250	126
Flounder, baked with butter	4 oz (114)	268	102
Haddock, fried	4 oz (114)	200	162

Food item	*Common Measure (Weight, g)*	*Sodium, mg*	*Calories*
	Fish and Seafood (cont)		
Halibut, broiled with butter	4 oz (114)	152	191
Lobster, boiled, meat only	4 oz (114)	183	123
Oysters, fresh	6 small—2 oz (58)	75	38
Salmon, broiled or baked with butter	4 oz (114)	133	207
Sardines, drained	1 can—3 1/4 oz (92)	598	187
Scallops, bay, steamed	10 to 12—4 oz (114)	302	153
Shrimp, raw	10 jumbo—3 oz (85)	137	98
Tuna, chunk, canned in oil, drained	1 can—3 1/4 oz (92)	328	182
Tuna, chunk, canned in water, drained	1 can—3 1/4 oz (92)	312	117
	Fruits		
Apple	1 medium (138)	2	118
Applesauce, sweetened	1/2 cup (125)	3	227
Apricots, canned, syrup	1/2 cup (129)	13	111
Apricots, dried	5 halves, medium (24)	2	62
Banana	1 medium (119)	2	68
Blackberries	1/2 cup (72)	1	42
Blueberries	1/2 cup (72)	1	45
Cantaloupe	1/2 melon (272)	24	47
Cherries, sweet, whole	1 cup (130)	2	82
Cherries, canned	1 cup (257)	10	110
Fruit cocktail, canned in syrup	1 cup (255)	15	195
Fruit cocktail, canned in water	1 cup (255)	15	95
Grapefruit	1/2 grapefruit (120)	1	26
Grapefruit, canned	1/2 cup (127)	2	89
Grapes	10 grapes (50)	1	23
Honeydew	1/5 melon (298)	28	61
Orange	1 medium (131)	1	47
Peach, skinned	1 medium (100)	1	29
Peaches, canned, syrup	1/2 cup (128)	8	100
Peaches, canned, water	1/2 cup (128)	8	38
Pear	1 medium (168)	1	93
Pears, canned, syrup	1/2 cup (128)	8	98
Pears, canned, water	1/2 cup (128)	8	40

Food item	Common Measure (Weight, g)	Sodium, mg	Calories
	Fruits (cont)		
Pineapple, fresh	1 cup (135)	1	71
Pineapple, canned, syrup	1 cup (255)	4	189
Pineapple, canned, water	1 cup (246)	4	96
Plums	10 plums (66)	1	30
Plums, canned, water	1 cup (256)	10	111
Prunes, cooked	1/2 cup (107)	4	108
Prunes, dried	5 prunes (43)	2	95
Raisins	1/4 cup, packed (36)	4	98
Rhubarb, cooked, sweetened	1/2 cup (135)	3	190
Strawberries	1/2 cup (75)	1	28
Strawberries, frozen, sweetened	1/2 cup (128)	1	139
Watermelon	1/16 melon (426)	8	55
	Meat and Poultry		
Bacon, regular	2 slices—1/2 oz (14)	274	61
Bacon, Canadian	1 slice—1 oz (28)	394	58
Bologna	1 slice (22)	224	61
Beef, corned	2 slices—3 oz (85)	802	315
Beef, fried, creamed	1 cup (245)	1,754	377
Beef, ground, lean	1 patty—4 oz (114)	76	249
Beef, lean, rump roast	2 slices—4 oz (114)	74	237
Beef, lean, round steak	6 oz (170)	180	444
Chicken, broiler	1/4 chicken (147)	58	120
Chicken, roasted	1/2 breast (98)	69	99
Chicken, fried	1 drumstick (56)	49	88
Frankfurter, all meat	1 frankfurter (57)	639	176
Ham, cured lean	2 slices—4 oz (114)	1,494	330
Ham, cured, country, lean	2 slices—4 oz (144)	980	304
Ham, fresh, lean	2 slices—4 oz (114)	79	426
Ham, chopped, lunchmeat	1 slice (21)	288	62
Ham, deviled	1 oz (28)	253	100
Lamb, loin chop, lean	2 chops—4 oz (114)	79	214
Lamb, leg, lean	2 slices—4 oz (114)	78	212
Liver, calf, fried	3 slices—4 oz (114)	133	298
Liver, chicken, simmered	5 livers—4 oz (114)	56	188

Food item	*Common Measure (Weight, g)*	*Sodium, mg*	*Calories*
	Meat and Poultry (cont)		
Liverwurst (braunschweiger)	1 slice (28)	324	88
Pork, loin roast, lean	1 slice—4 oz (114)	93	292
Salami, dry, beef and pork	1 slice (10)	226	45
Salami, cooked, beef and pork	1 slice (22)	255	88
Sausage, pork	1 link (13)	168	65
Sausage, pork	1 patty—2 oz (57)	259	129
Thuringer (summer sausage)	1 slice (22)	320	68
Turkey, dark meat	3 slices—4 oz (114)	91	218
Turkey, light meat	3 slices—4 oz (114)	61	200
Turkey, roll	1 oz (28)	166	70
Veal, cutlet, loin	1 cutlet—4 oz (114)	93	267
	Pasta		
Macaroni, plain, cooked	1 cup (140)	2	155
Macaroni with cheese	1 cup (200)	1,086	430
Pizza with cheese	1 slice—2 oz (57)	380	147
Pizza with sausage	1 slice—2 oz (57)	335	157
Spaghetti, with tomato sauce and cheese	1 cup (250)	955	190
Spaghetti, with tomato sauce, meatballs, and cheese	1 cup (248)	1,009	332
	Soups, Commercial Varieties, Condensed (Prepared With Addition of Equal Volumes of Water, Unless Noted)		
Bean	1 cup (250)	1,008	168
Beef broth	1 cup (241)	1,152	64
Chicken, cream of (with milk)	1 cup (245)	1,054	179
Chicken noodle	1 cup (240)	1,107	62
Chicken with rice	1 cup (241)	814	48
Clam chowder, Manhattan	1 cup (244)	938	81
Clam chowder, New England (with milk)	1 cup (248)	992	139
Minestrone	1 cup (241)	911	105
Mushroom, cream of (with milk)	1 cup (248)	992	216

Food item	Common Measure (Weight, g)	Sodium, mg	Calories
Soups, Commercial Varieties, Condensed (Prepared With Addition of Equal Volumes of Water, Unless Noted) (cont)			
Onion	1 cup (240)	1,051	65
Pea, green	1 cup (250)	987	130
Tomato	1 cup (245)	872	88
Tomato, cream of (with milk)	1 cup (250)	932	173
Turkey noodle	1 cup (240)	998	79
Vegetable beef	1 cup (245)	957	78
Vegetarian vegetable	1 cup (245)	823	78
Vegetables (Considered Fresh, Unless Listed Otherwise; Considered Cooked, Unless Indicated as Raw. Sodium Content of Cooked Vegetables is Content Before Salt is Added.)			
Artichoke	1 bud (120)	36	12
Asparagus	4 spears (60)	4	12
Asparagus, canned	4 spears (80)	298	17
Beans, baked, canned, with pork and tomato sauce	1/2 cup (145)	464	156
Beans, baked, canned, with pork and molasses sauce	1/2 cup (145)	303	192
Beans, green	1/2 cup (63)	3	16
Beans, green, canned	1/2 cup (65)	319	16
Beans, green, frozen	1/2 cup (68)	1	17
Beans, lima	1/2 cup (85)	1	95
Beans, lima, canned	1/2 cup (85)	228	82
Beans, lima, frozen	1/2 cup (85)	64	84
Beets	1/2 cup (85)	37	27
Beets, canned	1/2 cup (85)	240	42
Broccoli	1 stalk, medium (151)	18	39
Broccoli, frozen	1/2 cup (94)	18	24
Brussels sprouts	4 sprouts (84)	8	30
Brussels sprouts, frozen	1/2 cup (77)	8	26
Cabbage	1/2 cup (72)	8	16
Cabbage, raw	1/2 cup (35)	4	11
Carrots	1/2 cup (78)	26	34
Carrots, frozen	1/2 cup (113)	52	35
Carrots, raw	1 medium (72)	34	12
Cauliflower	1/2 cup (63)	6	14
Cauliflower, frozen	1/2 cup (90)	9	16
Cauliflower, raw	1/2 cup (58)	8	14

Food item	*Common Measure (Weight, g)*	*Sodium, mg*	*Calories*
Vegetables (Considered Fresh, Unless Listed Otherwise; Considered Cooked, Unless Indicated as Raw. Sodium Content of Cooked Vegetables is Content Before Salt is Added.) (cont)			
Celery, raw	1 stalk (20)	25	7
Corn	1 ear (140)	1	70
Corn, canned, creamed	1/2 cup (128)	336	105
Corn, canned, whole kernel	1/2 cup (83)	192	87
Cucumber, raw	6 large slices (28)	2	4
Lettuce, head, raw	1/4 head (135)	12	18
Lettuce, leaf, raw	1 cup (55)	5	10
Mushrooms	1/2 cup (35)	4	10
Okra	5 pods (53)	1	16
Onions, green, raw, with tops	2 medium (30)	2	14
Onions, raw	1 tbsp (10)	1	4
Peas, green	1/2 cup (80)	1	57
Peas, green, canned	1/2 cup (85)	247	82
Peas, green, frozen	1/2 cup (85)	106	55
Peppers, sweet	1/2 cup (75)	13	22
Pickles, dill	1 spear (30)	232	3
Pickles, sweet gherkin	1 whole pickle (15)	128	22
Potato, baked or boiled	1 medium (156)	5	145
Potatoes, french fried, unsalted	10 strips (50)	15	137
Potatoes, mashed, milk and salt added	1 cup (210)	632	137
Radishes, raw	5 medium (18)	8	7
Sauerkraut	1/2 cup (235)	777	21
Spinach, canned	1/2 cup (103)	455	25
Spinach, frozen	1/2 cup (50)	78	24
Spinach, raw	1/2 cup (55)	25	7
Squash, summer	1/2 cup (105)	3	13
Sweet potato, boiled	1 medium (132)	20	126
Sweet potato, canned	1 medium (100)	48	107
Tomato, raw	1 medium (123)	14	27
Tomatoes, canned	1/2 cup (120)	195	26
Snacks			
Caramels, plain or chocolate	1 oz (28)	74	113
Candy, milk chocolate	1 oz (28)	28	147

Food item	Common Measure (Weight, g)	Sodium, mg	Calories
	Snacks (cont)		
Corn chips, regular	1 oz (28)	231	157
Doughnuts, cake type, plain	1 doughnut (32)	160	125
Mints, chocolate-coated	1 small (11)	20	45
Nuts, cashews, dry-roasted, salted	4 tbsp—1 oz (28)	150	159
Peanut butter	1 tbsp—1 oz (16)	81	94
Peanuts, dry-roasted, salted	4 tbsp—1 oz (28)	123	166
Peanuts, roasted in oil, unsalted	4 tbsp—1 oz (28)	1	208
Popcorn, salted with butter	1 cup (9)	175	41
Popcorn, unsalted	1 cup (6)	1	23
Potato chips	14 chips—1 oz (28)	285	161
Pretzels, regular twist	5 pretzels—1/2 oz (14)	505	117

*Values calculated from US Department of Agriculture Home and Garden Bulletin 233, *The Sodium Content of Foods,* 1980, and USDA Agriculture Handbook No. 456, 1975, unless otherwise noted.

†Values do not include sodium contributed by the base water, which varies according to geographic location.

‡Values, provided by the National Soft Drink Association, are average and do not include sodium contributed by the base water, which varies according to geographic location.

§Data provided by cereal companies.

‖From USDA Agriculture Handbook 8-1, *Composition of Foods, Dairy Products and Egg Products, Raw, Processed, Prepared,* revised 1976.

¶From USDA Agriculture Handbook 8-4, *Composition of Foods, Fats and Oils, Raw, Processed, Prepared,* revised 1976.

#Cake and cookie values from USDA Handbook 8-1, revised 1976.

**Sodium value varies with different fruit flavorings.

Forty-five years ago, Dr. Walter Kempner demonstrated that a rice diet can control hypertension (and other diseases). He had his patients on 50 to 75 mg of salt per day. He observed that Oriental people use very little salt and that blood pressure problems are very rare in Asian countries.

A recent study demonstrated that infants whose salt is restricted for six weeks have lower blood pressure readings than infants who continue on regular feedings. Some people have an exquisite sensitivity to salt intake and swiftly elevate their blood pressures, while others have a better salt thermostat, so that the intake of sodium does not affect their blood pressure.

Along with weight loss and salt restriction, there is a push to control hypertension with relaxation techniques. If all of this fails, medications are used. The first line of drug therapy is the use of diuretics to loosen the salt content from the walls of the arteries through increasing the flow of urine. Diuretics are a safe group of medications. Side effects, such as occasional rash and sometimes worsening diabetes, are few. Potassium is lost from the body when some diuretics (like *Lasix* or *Hydrochlorothiazide*) are used and must be replaced. Very low potassium levels can cause serious consequences to the heart, like irregular heartbeats and even sudden death. The level of potassium in the blood has to be periodically checked. Other medications may be necessary, even pyramided one on the other, to attain a normal blood pressure of 135/85.

Beta-blockers are now very popular, followed by numerous other medications. In patients over the age of sixty, they are not as efficient in controlling blood pressure as they are in younger individuals.

There was recently a surprise finding that supplemental calcium ingestion can help to control blood pressure. Investigators at Cornell University Medical College are experimenting with the use of calcium to control mild hypertension. Diastolic blood pressure dropped significantly when calcium was administered. This finding needs to be confirmed before calcium supplements are included in the treatment of hypertension. These observations originated from the fact that patients who drink hard (that is, calcium-rich) water often have less hypertension.

Some of the major reasons that blood pressure is not

controlled are that the patient 1. does not take the medication as prescribed; 2. continues on a high-salt diet; 3. does not lose weight; and 4. does not have his blood pressure checked at a reasonable interval.

In 1985, there is little reason for hypertension not to be controlled. The patient needs, of course, to know if he has hypertension in the first place, and then he must have his blood pressure checked periodically, especially if there is a family history of it. The best way to avoid future bypass surgery and heart attacks is to have normal blood pressure. Throughout our country, there are health stations in which it can be kept track of.

5

The Medical Treatment of Angina

MEDICATIONS now available for the treatment of angina can effectively control the symptoms and may make bypass surgery unnecessary for most patients if combined with the other measures described.

Nitroglycerine

The workhorse drug for the treatment of angina is nitroglycerine. As we know, in large amounts this is a powerful explosive; the active ingredient of dynamite. Pure nitroglycerine is a heavy, oily liquid that is as clear as water and, when it explodes, expands to form gases that take up more than three times as much space as liquid. This magical compound was first discovered in 1846 by an Italian chemist, Dr. Ascani Sobrero. In 1864, Alfred Nobel, the Swedish chemist (who established the Nobel Prize for science, literature, and peace), obtained a patent for making nitroglycerine as an explosive, namely dynamite.

In 1844, Dr. Thomas Brunton experimented on the liquid form of nitroglycerine, called amyl nitrate. Thomas Brunton conceived angina to be caused by a paroxysmal increase in blood pressure, and amyl nitrate, he found, lowered the blood pressure and lessened the pain. (Today, amyl nitrate has earned the reputation of heightening the thrill of sexual activities; its street name is "poppers.") Nitroglycerine has now been used as an effective treatment for anginal attacks for some eighty years.

As we have seen, angina occurs through a simple supply and demand formula. If the heart demands oxygen and the supply cannot be delivered, then angina results. When the heart rate increases, or the blood pressure rises, the heart needs more oxygen. The body sends this message to the brain in the form of chest pain or angina.

Nitroglycerine is a safe medication. Occasionally, it causes a drop in blood pressure, which makes the patient feel weak and faint. The most annoying side effect is headache. Decreasing the dosage lessens the headache. In time, the headache will disappear; it can also be relieved with a mild analgesic such as aspirin. Nitroglycerine is available in tablets that are swallowed or placed under the tongue, or as a paste. The conventional way of administering nitroglycerine is under the tongue. It is generally stored in a tinted glass vial because it is sensitive to light and loses its strength rapidly after several months. Patients will sometimes experience a burning sensation as they place the pill under the tongue, but this assures them that the pill is still active. A positive response should occur in several minutes.

Nitroglycerine can also be swallowed; it is absorbed through the intestine, but part of it is inactivated by the liver. That is the reason why the medication given under the tongue is much more rapid and effective. The most effective and popular method of administering nitroglycerine is through the skin, commonly through a "patch." (For centuries, there have been attempts to give medications through the skin through the use of rubs, liniments, ointments, and topical preparations, but almost all of these earlier efforts were ineffective and caused serious reactions.)

In 1963, dynamite workers exposed to nitroglycerine experienced strange effects, such as flushing, headaches, and weakness. This was because nitroglycerine was being absorbed through the skin. The workers provided the clue for the preparation of ointments of nitroglycerine. The ointment, however, had problems; it was difficult to measure the amount of medication or the rate of delivery. Further, the nitroglycerine paste had to be covered up in order to prevent evaporation, and it was a nuisance to change the paste every four hours. Then came the transdermal form of nitroglycerine, the so-called patch. These patches are like Band-Aids containing chemicals with nitroglycerine. The nitroglycerine is slowly released from the stick-on patch through the skin and into the blood. There are numerous preparations of the patch or disc, such as Transderm-Nitro, Nitro-Dur, and Nitrodisc. Nitroglycerine is released at a certain rate per hour, and at the end of twenty-four hours, most of the drug is used up. The paste or the transderm patches can be placed anywhere on the body. They do not have to be placed on the chest to be near the heart, but may be placed on the thighs or on the arms. The area of placement should be changed regularly as some patients develop a rash.

Transdermal delivery of nitroglycerine is for the prevention of angina attacks, not for an acute attack; unlike the fast-acting pill, it takes thirty minutes for the nitroglycerine in the patch to have its effect. The level of nitroglycerine drops within a half hour after the patch is removed. It may be necessary for increasingly potent patches to be used, from 5 mg to 10 mg and even 20 mg. There are different patterns of absorption in patients, and some people need more and others less.

Nitroglycerine taken sublingually (placed under the tongue) is extraordinarily effective for treatment of an acute attack of angina. In addition, if there are certain activities which bring on an anginal attack, it might be worthwhile to use the nitroglycerine prophylactically, that is, in anticipation of an attack. For example, some patients develop anginal symptoms prior to and during sexual intercourse, and it is worthwhile to give nitroglycerine before the attack. Others develop anginal symptoms while they are walking a short distance, or in the cold weather, or even before meals. Some patients develop angina as soon as they lie down quietly at night. In all these cases, taking nitroglycerine prophylactically is beneficial; however, angina can usually be controlled by increasing the dosage of the patch. If not enough nitroglycerine is given, angina may persist. For example, a patch of 5 mg may be insufficient and 10 mg should be used.

Case: Before transdermal nitroglycerine had appeared on the scene, a sixty-two-year-old bank manager developed severe chest pain classical of coronary artery disease. A stress test and thallium stress test confirmed the diagnosis. For reasons to be described later, the only medication that he could use safely was nitroglycerine and calcium channel blockers. He took several preparations of nitroglycerine that were swallowed, and he took others under the tongue. He increased the nitroglycerine tablets by mouth to four and the nitroglycerine under his tongue to every three hours. He was taking up to twenty nitroglycerine tablets per day. He tolerated this well, and his chest pain subsided completely. He was advised to have cardiac catheterization and bypass surgery, which he refused. Five years later, he switched to the Transderm patches in addition to his pills, and he remains symptom-free. During one of his chest pain examinations, an electrocardiogram demonstrated specific changes diagnostic of coronary artery spasms; nitroglycerine is also particularly useful for this condition (as are the channel calcium blockers, discussed below).

Comment: If he had not increased the nitroglycerine dosage, he certainly would have eventually had bypass surgery. He also went on a strict dietary program, lowering his cholesterol level to 180, only about 40 percent of his pre-treatment level. Included in his treatment was a cholestyramine bile salt to lower his cholesterol, coupled with a moderate exercise program. It has been years since his rejection of the bypass surgery and he remains comfortable. He has not sustained a heart attack, and the quality of his life is suitable enough for him, even though he does have to take many pills and continues the patches.

Headaches are both common and annoying when nitroglycerine is taken in any form. Unfortunately, some patients refuse to take nitroglycerine preparations because of the severity of the headaches. Most of the time, however, the headaches subside after a certain period of time and can be relieved by taking a mild analgesic, such as Tylenol (acetaminophen) or aspirin. Some patients have an undue sensitivity to nitroglycerine and their blood pressure can drop. This is primarily a nuisance problem because it causes the patient to feel weak and woozy upon standing. Nitroglycerine is best taken when sitting down, and the patient should then remain seated for some minutes.

I also prefer that patients not suddenly stop taking nitroglycerine after using it for many years, because there may be a reflex constriction of the arteries and angina may reappear. It was discovered that after many years of exposure to nitroglycerine in manufacturing plants, workers who changed jobs developed episodes of chest pain.

During a heart attack, if patients continue having chest pain, nitroglycerine is given intravenously to relieve the pain and possibly also lessen the severity of the heart attack by decreasing the amount of oxygen demand and increasing the oxygen supply, through lowering the blood pressure. As a rule, intravenous nitroglycerine will control the chest pain and make it unnecessary to rush into cardiac catheterization and from there to bypass surgery.

Beta-Blockers

Beta-blockers (or B-blockers) are a remarkable class of medications that decrease the oxygen demand on the heart by blocking the sympathetic nervous system, which forms different chemicals, like adrenaline. As a result of the blockage, the blood pressure is lowered, the heart rate drops, and the pulse slows. The beta-blocker also reduces the ability of the heart to contract.

In order for the beta-blockers to be effective, the pulse rate has to be lowered to between fifty and sixty beats per minute. If the pulse rate increases under stress, or with minimal physical activity, such as climbing stairs, then that patient is not receiving an adequate dosage to relieve the symptoms.

It is imperative that beta-blockers be carefully administered, especially in patients who have a history of congestive heart failure (or severe bronchial asthma).

The physician checks the pulse rate each time he sees the patient and also teaches the patient to take his own pulse rate. An acceptable pulse rate to achieve is approximately sixty beats per minute. A simple way to measure the efficacy of a slowing pulse rate is to have the patient jump up and down on one foot, or to engage in bending exercises; if the heart rate before taking the drug is 120 beats per minute and remains at that rate after two minutes of this type of effort, then the patient is not receiving an adequate dosage. The exercise response should be brought down by approximately 50 percent, to a pulse rate of sixty. If the expected heart rate response is not achieved, it can mean the drug has not been taken, or that it has not been absorbed, or that it is being deactivated by the liver.

Unfortunately, as good as beta-blockers are, they do cause annoying side effects. Impotence can occur. Fatigue may also be a problem, which at times becomes intolerable and frightening to the patient. Depression and fatigue may make the patient feel worse than his angina did. Some patients believe that the fatigue and the exhaustion originate from their disease and that the end is near. Sometimes the patient just cannot tolerate beta-blockers. Another alternative is the channel calcium blockers.

Case: After her angina had been adequately controlled with nitroglycerine and beta-blockers (and beta-blockers are often given together with nitroglycerine to help correct the two reasons for angina: oxygen lack with oxygen requirement), a fifty-eight-year-old woman confronted her physician with the simple statement, "I think I'm dying." She went on to tell the physician how the slightest effort exhausted her, that she no longer had the will to live because her fatigue was utterly unbearable. The alert physician decreased the beta-blocker medication and she gradually began to improve, and when he switched her to another preparation, her fatigue disappeared entirely, and she has become an optimistic and active woman. (When patients have the feeling that they are getting worse, it is very important that they tell the physician.)

When the heart muscle contracts weakly, fluid can back up into the lungs, causing shortness of breath or congestive heart failure. Congestive heart failure is worsened by beta-blockers, and in some instances, when the heart is not functioning properly, beta-blockers can push an individual into congestive heart failure. All treatments must be individualized, and the physician will adjust the dosage according to each person's height, weight, and age. Some older patients tolerate beta-blockers poorly, and they are more likely to suffer heart failure.

Some patients receiving beta-blockers develop marked slowing of their pulse and a drop in blood pressure, resulting in dizziness. Indeed, one of the other uses of this medication is for the treatment of hypertension, or high blood pressure.

Beta-blockers maintain a low blood pressure and pulse rate. The sudden withdrawal of the medication causes a sharp rise in the pulse rate and in the blood pressure. The heart now has a greater demand for oxygen, and since the supply is not increased, the patient can suffer a heart attack. Beta-blockers must be reduced slowly, and only under the direction of a physician.

Often patients ask, "Can I exercise if I'm taking beta-blockers?" The answer is a qualified Yes.

I have known tennis players who, after their heart attacks, continued taking beta-blockers and nitroglycerine, and as they became fully rehabilitated after two years, gradually decreased them to the point where they are now very active without any medication.

I am often asked, "Do I have to take this medication forever?" The answer is that "nothing is forever." Many patients, once they become completely rehabilitated, with proper weight loss, a low-cholesterol diet, and the cessation of smoking, will find they can gradually decrease their medications.

Today, patients with mild or moderate angina who are medically treated do as well as surgically treated patients. If the mild angina becomes severe angina, then they become candidates for surgery. Coronary bypass surgery can often be avoided if the patient is willing to continue taking medications in adequate amounts.

Case: A fifty-eight-year-old man was diagnosed as having coronary artery disease and angina. He was taking nitroglycerine paste and a beta-blocker medication. His angina continued and his physician advised him to have bypass surgery. The patient consulted another physician for an opinion. The physical examination disclosed a man with a blood pressure of 160/110; his weight was 190, and he was 5′6″ tall. The heart examination was normal, except that the resting pulse rate was 80. When the patient exercised, by jumping on one foot, the pulse rate climbed to 120 and remained there after he stopped, for the next ten minutes. When the dosage of the beta-blocker was increased, the resting pulse leveled at 60 and jumped little upon exercise. His angina was controlled.

Can beta-blockers prevent heart attacks? There is some indirect evidence that they cut down the possibility of heart attack by their effect on controlling the blood pressure and lowering the pulse rate. A study at the Glasgow Blood Pressure Clinic noted that "there was a highly significant tendency for men and women who were taking beta-blockers to suffer fewer heart attacks and strokes" than patients taking other forms of treatment. And there is clear evidence that beta-blockers decrease the chances of a second heart attack.

Calcium Channel Blocking Drugs

A new class of exciting drugs, calcium channel blockers, has finally been approved by the Food and Drug Administration (FDA). These drugs have been available in Europe for at least ten years. Their use may change the entire face of coronary artery disease. Angina, as we have seen, may result from spasm of the coronary arteries, a spasm that may be superimposed on an artery that is blocked. Spasm of the coronary arteries may be a significant factor in the onset of a heart attack. It has been approximated that 93 percent of patients with chest pain at rest have spasm of the coronary arteries, although it is frequently difficult to prove that this is the cause of the pain. These drugs act to reduce calcium uptake by the heart and smooth muscles of the coronary arteries. There are high complex mechanisms why calcium in the wall of the artery can cause spasm. Studies are underway to discover the real role of calcium. The effect is to reduce and eliminate spasm of the coronary arteries. There are three different types of calcium blockers now available: *Nifedipine*, *Verapamil*, and *Diltiazem.* Each has its own characteristics and needs to be tailored for that individual; for example, in some patients, Nifedipine sometimes causes the angina to get worse.

When patients who are suffering from mild angina are not improving with beta-blockers and nitroglycerine, calcium channel blockers should be added to the program before a decision is made to send the patient to coronary bypass surgery. All the studies performed on the medical control of mild angina have demonstrated that medical therapy is as good as the surgical treatment to prevent heart attacks and prolong life. These studies, however, did not include the new channel calcium blockers. Many cardiologists feel that with the addition of channel calcium blockers, it will be shown that the medical treatment will be superior to surgical treatment in most cases of mild and moderate angina.

Each of the channel calcium blockers has side effects. It is important, when they are added to beta-blockers, that their interactions be considered and the dosage carefully adjusted. For example, the addition of Verapamil to a beta-blocker can put the patient into congestive heart failure if the heart is functioning weakly. It is always best for the patient to consult his physician about the interaction of drugs.

A Boston cardiologist, Dr. Eugene Braunwald, has been quoted as saying, "They are almost too good to be true." He may well be right.

Table 3. Drug interactions

Medication	*Reaction*	*Recommendation*
Verapamil plus propranolol	Cardiac failure, hypotension, cardiac conduction abnormalities	Avoid giving combination to patients with poor heart function
Diltiazem plus B-blocker	Probably similar to Verapamil and Nifedipine	Follow recommendations for Verapamil and Nifedipine
Clonidine plus propranolol	Severe rebound hypertension when clonidine is withdrawn in the presence of B-blockade	Discontinue B-blocker therapy before clonidine is tapered

Vitamin E: Does It Help?

The vitamin E story began in 1922 when two doctors named Evans and Bishop discovered that this vitamin was needed by female rats to reproduce and was also an essential compound for birds and other animals. Vitamin E deficiency has been reported in some African children who are severely malnourished and in patients suffering from malabsorption and other rare conditions.

The average American diet contains about 16 mg per day of vitamin E. It has been calculated that two to five units of vitamin E are needed to prevent the breakdown of red blood cells in children. Sixty-four percent of vitamin E is derived from oils and fats, fruits and vegetables; egg yolk and meat contain small amounts. The advocates of vitamin supplements state that food processing destroys vitamin E. While it is true that there is some loss, it is not serious.

If you eat a normal diet, you ingest ample amounts of vitamin E. The excitement over vitamin E occurred with Dr. Alfred Shute's theory, based on a chance observation by his brother, that a patient who was receiving a wheat germ product orally for another reason enjoyed complete relief of angina pectoris. Dr. Shute and his associates concluded that it was the vitamin E content of the wheat germ that helped relieve the symptoms of angina, and also that the arteriosclerosis of the arteries of the legs and veins benefited. They state that they have treated more than 30,000 heart patients and that "the medical profession has wasted a twenty-year search for a drug that already exists." They say that the epidemic of angina that plagues the United States occurred after 1910 because of the decreased vitamin E in our diet. They reject all other theories, such as high cholesterol, cigarette smoking, inactivity and diabetes. Such thinking, as we shall now see, is almost certainly wrong and dangerous.

Some patients with angina have a spontaneous remission; that is, the chest pain disappears entirely without any treatment. In fact, there is a large psychological component in the treatment of angina, called the *placebo effect.* If we administer an empty capsule and tell the patient it will relieve his chest pain, symptoms will disappear in a certain percentage of patients.

Placebo dates back to the earliest times of treatment of medical conditions. It has been said that most treatment used in medieval days was placebo. Quacks thrive on the placebo effect in a person—the power of suggestion is so strong that a worthless medication will have its effect if the doctor is convincing enough.

Dexedrine, a well-known stimulating drug of the nervous system, was given to a group of subjects who were told they were testing a sleeping pill. Nearly three-quarters of the patients did go to sleep! The same groups were given placebo pills (cellulose) and were told the pills would keep them awake for twenty-four hours. Again, three-quarters could not fall asleep for forty-eight hours.

Placebo, in my opinion, should not be used for the treatment of an illness. Pitifully, patients seek out medical care for terminal chronic illnesses from quacks who peddle chemically worthless pills.

According to Dr. Shute, the beneficial effects of vitamin E derive from its anti-clotting power and its ability to open the diseased artery. He claims that a patient treated with the appropriate amounts of vitamin E (namely, ten to forty times the amounts specified in the recommended dietary allowance) can avoid clots of the legs as well as clots of the lung.

Coronary artery disease, however, is not a new condition that suddenly appeared when we began to eat white bread; moreover, the American diet has not been shown to be deficient in vitamin E. Our present diet actually has increased amounts of vitamin E. Vitamin E seems to have little, if any, beneficial effect on the patient with coronary artery disease. Similar statements can be made about the beneficial effects of vitamin C in preventing coronary artery disease. Large dosages of vitamin C were given to patients with high levels of cholesterol and there were no beneficial effects.

The vitamin advocates and self-styled nutritionists urge use of vitamin E to prevent the following: coronary artery disease, arteriosclerosis of the lower legs (peripheral vascular disease), clots of the legs, thrombophlebitis, leg cramps, fibrocystic breast disease, complications of diabetes, sterility, and the aging process.

Nutritionist writers are quoted as saying that vitamin E is the "granddaddy" of all vitamins because "it puts oxygen quality in each blood cell." The facts are as follows: vitamin E seems to prolong the life span of red blood cells exposed to the sun or to violet rays; it has also been reported in the

New England Journal of Medicine that it possibly benefits infants who have congenital enzyme deficiency and some rare lung abnormalities.

None of the studies have provided us with evidence that vitamin E will prevent or treat angina or arteriosclerosis. There is no evidence that it will make bypass surgery unnecessary. Although vitamin E has been reported to be safe, I am strongly in favor of not taking excessive amounts, because it is not innocuous. From a study performed at the Mannow Research Laboratory, at the Palm Beach Institute of Medical Research, and from dozens of other legitimate reviews by the *Journal of the American Medical Association* and the *New England Journal of Medicine*, it is clear that excessive amounts of vitamin E have been reported to: 1. increase the level of cholesterol; 2. cause abnormalities of hormones and blood cells; and 3. alter metabolism. Further, a list of dozens of other possible complications associated with vitamin E is reported in the *Journal of American Medicine* (July 1981), as follows: 1. phlebitis; 2. embolism; 3. hypertension; 4. fatigue; 5. vaginal bleeding; 6. headache; 7. dizziness; 8. nausea, diarrhea, and intestinal cramps; 9. aggravation of angina; 10. aggravation of diabetes; 11. disturbances of reproduction; 12. slowed rate of healing; 13. chapping of lips; 14. visual complaints—the list goes on and on.

In conclusion, I do not advocate vitamin E as a form of prevention of arteriosclerosis until further studies come to light, and I urge patients to desist from excessive amounts, which may include megadoses of 800 to 1,600 units. I look forward to proof of the alleged benefits of vitamin E. Such proof does not now exist.

Aspirin

Acetylsalicylic acid, the chemical name for aspirin, is an ancient medication dating back 2,000 years, since Hippocrates' time, and has been used for the treatment of pain throughout the centuries. It is derived from the willow leaves, as well as from many other shrubs, such as jasmine-madder. The North American Indian tribes used it as a fever-reducer, and the aborigines called Hottentots, of South Africa, used it for pain. Its many known uses are legion.

The actual active ingredient was developed in the laboratories of Friedrich Bayer and Company. It was Dr. Felix Hoffmann, a young research chemist, who refined its use in the course of looking for a remedy for his crippled father, who was suffering from severe rheumatoid arthritis. After doing his own research, he carried his notes to the Bayer Company's director of pharmacological research, Dr. Heinrich Dreser, and it was Dreser who labeled the product "aspirin." They found that it was an extraordinary drug—one that we are just beginning to really appreciate in 1985.

In the United States, we take some 12,000 tons of aspirin per year. The use of aspirin has increased since it was recommended in some medical studies as a form of prevention for heart attack, strokes, and lung embolism. Aspirin actually works by interfering with the platelets sticking together—like chewing gum on a chair: the first step in forming a clot. The reduction of an enzyme called *prostacycline* prevents the platelets from sticking together. Increase of the enzyme does the opposite.

There is some strong and convincing data that by preventing the platelets from sticking together, aspirin may prevent heart attacks. The question is, how much aspirin should be taken? There has been a great deal of controversy in this regard. The consensus at the present time is that one 325-mg aspirin every day is adequate to prevent clotting. When a patient is admitted into a coronary care unit and chest pain continues (unstable angina), giving several aspirins a day diminishes the death rate by 30 to 40 percent.

On the whole, aspirin is a safe drug (indeed, many cardiologists take one aspirin per day). The side effects are well known. Occasionally, it does cause gastrointestinal bleeding and it certainly should not be given to any person who has an ulcer or even a history of ulcer. Most recently, the combination of aspirin and *dipyridamole (Persantine)* has been used to prevent bypass grafts from closing. Aspirin and Persantine given before surgery, and then continued for one year after the operation, cause a marked reduction in graft closure.

In a multicenter trial conducted by the Veterans' Administration Cooperative Study, reported in the *New England Journal of Medicine* (May 1983), a single dose of 325 mg aspirin was given for twelve weeks to 1,266 men who had unstable angina—angina that continues and is a forerunner of a heart attack. The progression of the angina to a heart attack or death was reduced 51 percent in the patients who received aspirin. It was recommended by these investigators that aspirin should be added for the management of angina.

Sudden death can result from a clot forming in the arteries during the first hours of a heart attack. In another article in the *New England Journal of Medicine* (May 1984), it was reported that seventy-four of one hundred patients who died had a thrombus (clot) in the coronary artery. I advise my patients who have no ulcer disease to quickly take one-half aspirin at the onset of an angina attack.

EDTA Chelation Therapy

Unfortunately, when our medical treatment fails, patients sometimes rush for other alternatives to treat their angina. This reaction is reminiscent of arthritis patients who wear copper bracelets, sit in uranium mines, and go to Mexico to arthritis clinics where they ingest plant roots. A form of unproven treatment that has become rather popular throughout this country is EDTA (ethylene-diaminetetracetic acid) chelation therapy. Three grams of EDTA are given one to four times a week, at a cost ranging from $60 to $110 per infusion. The efficacy of this form of treatment has been reported, in particular, in the *Journal of Holistic Medicine.* Thousands of patients have received chelation therapy and many claim freedom from angina. However, the American College of Cardiology has not been able, as of the present time, to evaluate this form of treatment.

EDTA has been in use in medicine for at least forty years for the removal of calcium deposits. Reports of its use by the Russians and the Czechoslovakians, as well as in New Zealand, claim that EDTA removes calcium from the arterial wall. In one study, rabbits who had marked arteriosclerosis were placed on a low-cholesterol diet for twenty-three weeks and then received EDTA treatment. The calcified plaques disappeared. However, similar experiments have been done on rabbits where the cholesterol deposits disappeared without EDTA treatment, simply by modifying the diet. EDTA treatment has also been used for Alzheimer's disease on the assumption that there is an excessive amount of aluminum in the brain in patients with this illness. Chelation was first synthesized in Germany in 1930 and was used to treat lead poisoning.

The people who give chelation therapy admit that the patients who are receiving it stop smoking and go on a strict dietary program. The EDTA administrators claim that the mechanism of action is not understood. They further claim that it does not cause the kidney function to deteriorate, as had been alleged (an FDA panel, headed by Dr. David Spence in 1970, reported thirteen patients died from chelation therapy as a result of kidney failure). It is reported that almost a thousand physicians are using this form of treatment.

I am waiting to see a good controlled study to convince

me that chelation therapy is of benefit to the patient. As mentioned before, placebo is a wonderful form of treatment, and it has been known since the beginning of recorded time that patients' pain can be eased with medications that have no active ingredients. I would be using chelation therapy today in my clinical practice if there was enough evidence to show that it indeed helps angina; it certainly would be another tool to avoid bypass surgery.

According to the American Academy of Medical Prevention, there are 300,000 patients who have been treated with chelation therapy. But insurance companies do not pay for this therapy because it is not an approved form of treatment.

Case: Mrs. R.K. is an overweight fifty-seven-year-old female who suffers from diabetes and hypertension. She has had a long-standing history of angina and eventually suffered a heart attack. Her symptoms continued after her discharge from the hospital and it was decided that she would have cardiac catheterization, which disclosed widespread disease of her anterior descending coronary artery. Her heart showed a great deal of enlargement and she was not a good candidate for surgery because her arteries were diffusely narrowed. Subsequently, she was placed on a vigorous diet, predominantly containing vegetables and fish, and on beta-blocker medication, which slowed her pulse to 50; a channel blocker was added, including an ample amount of nitropaste. Mrs. R.K. became symptom-free, with some periodic episodes of chest pain.

Comment: On her own, this patient decided to search out someone who prescribes chelation therapy. I did not discourage her from doing this and followed her situation for the next three and a half months. She in turn continued with her medications, and her diabetes was well controlled, as was her hypertension. She periodically appeared in the office complaining of some shortness of breath, particularly after her chelation therapy had been given. (I learned that the salt content of the product she was receiving might possibly contribute to increasing shortness of breath.) Her chest pain remained under control, and she definitely stated that she felt better, but she would not admit that perhaps the diet was playing an important role, as well as the medication and the psychological effect of having something done on a weekly basis. In either case, I tried to discourage her from continuing her treatment, but to no avail. It seems likely that any lessening of her illness would be due primarily to her continuing with previously prescribed medication, a strict dietary program, and low cholesterol, and having a general feeling of well-being.

6

Exercise and Your Heart

"EXERCISE ferments the humors, casts them into their proper channels, throws off redundancies, and helps nature know secret distributions without which the body cannot subsist in its vigor, nor the soul act with cheerfulness."

Since the beginning of time, exercise has served as a form of recreation and has promoted a general state of well-being. Among other exercises, the ancient Egyptians and Greeks ran long distances, rode horses, wrestled, dove into ice-cold water, and climbed mountains. There is no doubt that when you engage in a regular form of physical activity, you feel better, but does it do anything for the heart?

It wasn't too long ago that a patient diagnosed as having angina or any heart problem was advised by his physician to cease all strenuous activity. Patients who sustained a heart attack were often hospitalized for six weeks at a time, with no activity. Complete abstinence from physical exertion was advocated and anginal patients were confined to bed, sometimes for six months to a year. Even today I see patients who have been advised to eliminate all forms of exercise and physical activity. Surely, there *are* certain cardiac conditions, such as a seriously diseased aortic valve, when the patient should not exercise.

Dr. Paul Dudley White always said that exercise is the best tranquilizer; when he took leave of his friends, he never said, "Take it easy"; rather, he said, "Take it hard." There is the classic story of Clarence Demar, who participated in marathon races early in this century. When he died from an accident, an autopsy revealed that his coronary arteries were, most beneficially, two to three times normal size.

The decade of the eighties might be looked upon as the exercise age. There are bicycling, jogging, and cross-country skiing. The Boston marathon, which is in its eighty-eighth year, attracts thousands of runners, as does the New York marathon. Yet Neil Armstrong, the famous astronaut, was once quoted as saying that he rarely exercised because he has only so many heartbeats in a lifetime and he doesn't want to waste any of his. On the other hand, Satchel Paige, that most famous and witty pitcher, advised us to "keep the juices dangling."

Dr. Richard Ackstein, in 1957, demonstrated that animals, after an induced heart attack, formed new blood vessels when they exercised. It is now firmly established, after numerous observations and studies, that exercise is beneficial, and that a lack of exercise appears to shorten life and to predispose to heart attacks. Dr. Jerry Morris, who examined 31,000 London Transport employees, ages thirty-five to sixty-four, noted that the more sedentary bus drivers had 1.5 times more coronary artery disease than active conductors who spent most of their day going up and down the steps of a double-decker bus. The drivers had higher blood pressures and cholesterol levels than the conductors.

Similar studies have shown that former Harvard football players had fewer heart attacks if they continued their exercising. Records of 172 Harvard and Yale graduates who had been members of the crew squad between the years 1882 and 1902 were investigated. The average life span of the crew members was sixty-seven years, which was significantly greater than the average control, which was sixty years. Dr. Ralph Paffenberger reported a twenty-two-year follow-up study on San Francisco longshoremen. Three hundred men were studied who were twenty-five to sixty-four years old. The workers were divided into two levels of work activity. The less active group had a 30 percent higher coronary death rate than the more active group.

What are the effects of a lot of exercise on the heart? The athlete has a lower pulse rate, and the blood pressure is lower. In the animal world, experiments have shown that chronic exercise enlarges the hearts. Wild animals have larger hearts than domestic animals. Exercise rats have larger blood vessels.

Besides lowering blood pressure, exercise tends to help to maintain a lowered cholesterol and elevates the high-density lipoprotein. Patients who regularly exercise tend to have less fatigue, better sleeping patterns, less depression, than those who do not. Some men who regularly exercise report increased sexual abilities. Although exercise has not been shown to slow the progression of arteriosclerosis, people who are more physically fit have a greater chance of preventing a heart attack, avoiding the need for coronary bypass surgery, and living longer, especially when they simultaneously control blood pressure and cholesterol intake. High levels of HDL are found in marathon runners (and I have previously noted how HDL is a protective mechanism on the heart). Obesity is a prime promoter of atherosclerosis, diabetes, and hypertension. People who exercise, as a rule, are not fat.

It is important to understand that the amount of exercise each person should undertake for prevention, or after developing angina, or after a heart attack, is an individual matter and should be prescribed. No one over the age of forty should take up a strenuous exercise program before consulting a physician.

The purpose of the exercise is to allow the heart to work more efficiently so that its demand for oxygen is minimal and the availability of oxygen is maximal. This can be achieved by converting the heart into an even more efficient pump. When it can eject blood voluminously with the least expenditure of energy, that is, with a low pulse rate and a low blood pressure, the heart can achieve its maximum efficiency. A heart that reaches a blood pressure of 220 and a pulse of 180 with minimal exercise is not an efficiently working heart.

An Exercise Prescription

The exercise prescription of Dr. William B. Kannel, who heads the Framingham studies, a twenty-year ongoing investigation, follows:

1. It should be at least three times a week, or, better yet, four or five times a week.
2. The exercise should be approximately of twenty minutes' duration, and it should be continuous.
3. The exercise should be one that gives the patient pleasure and enjoyment.
4. Exercise should be fun and should not be a chore.

Dr. Kannel states that the intensity of exercise should be 60 to 80 percent of the maximal heart rate reserve. Subtract the patient's age from 220 and then take 60, 70, or 80 percent of that figure as the heart rate at which the patient should exercise. For example, a fifty-year-old man was prescribed an exercise heart-rate goal of 136 beats per minute after he was tested on a stress test.

No exercise program should be started in any person over forty, expecially one who has angina, unless a cardiac stress test is performed to determine what safe level the pulse rate may reach. I recommend that any patient with heart disease who starts an exercise program stop smoking, be on a weight-reduction program if indicated, and have his blood pressure controlled with adequate medications. Ideally, an exercise program should expend approximately 1,500 to 2,000 calories a week. This can be achieved, for example, by jogging ten miles a week at a relatively slow pace. The exercise should be started gradually, with a warmup and stretching period, and should be regulated, by the patient, according to the pulse rate at which chest pain appears. For example, if chest pain appears when the pulse rate reaches 120, the exercise program should be designed to reach a pulse rate of 110. For those patients who are non-athletic and who have no desire to do any form of exercise, the simplest thing to do is to jog in place for several minutes a day, counting the pulse and gradually increasing the exercise time each week. The patient is then re-tested with the exercise stress test, and if there are no abnormal changes, he is encouraged to continue this jogging program. By the end of fifty weeks he should be jogging one to two miles at home every week. The exercise is conducted before meals, and never when the patient is ill. If the daily jogging is too fatiguing, it should be performed every other day. Swimming can be substituted for jogging.

Isometric exercise benefits muscles but does little for the heart. Isometric exercises consist of weight-lifting types of exercise, in contrast to such *isotonic* exercises as swimming. All good exercise programs recommend that the pulse be taken prior to the exercise and immediately after. After a one-minute jog, a pulse rate between 85 and 100 is usual. This can vary according to the individual. At the end of a year, exercise that results in a pulse of 120 or 130 is acceptable. A pulse rate of 150 after a minor walk or minor exercise needs to be reported to the physician. If you jog in place for three minutes and your pulse reaches 140, then you must cease jogging three minutes and start again later at a one-minute level.

The amount of calories that one uses in each exercise will depend on each person's weight. A 170-pound man who is running in place for 90 counts per minute will use up 275 calories per hour. A 196-pound man who is running in place at 90 counts per minute will be using 380 calories.

A stationary bicycle is also extraordinarily useful. The boredom of using it can be alleviated by placing it in front of a television set and watching a favorite program. Under no circumstances should exercise be performed immediately after eating a meal, or if there is fatigue, or a cold or other illness. Exercise should be discontinued if it causes chest pain, weakness, or dizziness.

The most beneficial forms of exercise for the heart are jogging, swimming, and bicycling. The least effective are the isometrics—weightlifting, chinning, sit-ups, and so on.

An exercise prescription should be based on the patient's performance on a treadmill test or bicycle. If a person's maximum tolerance is measured on a treadmill as ten *mets* (one met is the metabolic equivalent of 3.5 milliliters of oxygen per one gram per minute at rest), the exercise prescription is 70 percent of this value, or seven mets. Seven mets include jogging slowly at approximately five miles per hour, cycling twelve miles per hour, swimming one mile per hour, square dancing, and tennis. This corresponds to the bicycle stress test, approximately fifteen calories per minute. Other physical activity energy expenditures are listed on table 1.

The major problem arising from an exercise program is musculoskeletal: painful joints and backs and sprained ankles. Joggers sustain injuries to their calves and knees from the repeated jolt on these joints. Patients with back problems can aggravate their ailment with jogging. Tennis players develop painful elbows that can take months to improve. Each person, before engaging in sports like tennis, jogging, or racquetball, should be knowledgeable regarding proper warmups prior to the exercise. Stretching joints is essential to try to avoid rupture of muscles, like the Achilles tendon. Rupture can cause prolonged anguish and disability.

The exercise program must be coupled with a strict dietary regulation. In the majority of patients who exercise, the heart work (the ejection fraction) markedly improves, the blood pressure is well controlled, the cholesterol level is decreased, and the patient regains control of his own life—the best treatment for fear.

Below are the energy requirements of common daily activities, based on a 185-pound man. The caloric requirement can be calculated by multiplying the ideal weight of the person by 10. A female with an ideal weight of 130 requires 1,300 calories a day. Measured in calories per hour and mets.

Table 4. Energy requirements of common daily activities

Activity	*Cal/Hr*	*Mets*	*Work Activities*	*Cal/Hr*	*Mets*
Conversation	85	1	Lawn mowing (power mower)	250	3.5
Dressing/undressing	140	2			
Driving an automobile	150	2	Lawn mowing (hand)	465	6.5
Eating	85	1	Bricklaying	240	3.5
Showering	250	3.5	Carpentry	400	5.5
Sitting	75	1	Felling trees	480	6.5
Standing, relaxed	85	1	Gardening	200–300	3.4
Washing hands/face	150	2	Plastering	245	3.5

Activity	*Cal/Hr*	*Mets*	*Work Activities*	*Cal/Hr*	*Mets*
Wheelchair propulsion	150	2	Shoveling (hand)	400–500	5.5–6.5
Resting, supine	60	1	Tending furnace	620	8.5
			Tractor plowing	250	3.5
			Wood chopping or sawing	400	5.5

Housework	*Cal/Hr*	*Mets*	*Recreation/ Sports*	*Cal/Hr*	*Mets*
Cleaning windows	220	3	Bowling	260	3.5
Hand sewing	85	1	Canoeing 2.5 mph	200	3
Hand-washing clothes	180	2.5	Cycling 5.5 mph	250	3.5
Hanging wash	270	3.5	Cycling 12 mph	660	9
Ironing, standing	250	3.5	Dancing	330	4.5
Kneading dough	200	2.5	Golfing	300	4
Machine sewing	110	1.5	Horseback riding (trotting)	400	5.5
Making beds	235	3			
Mopping	250	3.5	Jogging 10 mph	900	13
Peeling potatoes	175	2.5	Painting, sitting	120	1.5
Polishing furniture	145	2	Playing piano	150	2

Housework	*Cal/Hr*	*Mets*	*Recreation/ Sports*	*Cal/Hr*	*Mets*
Scrubbing floor	215	3	Roller skating	350	5
Scrubbing, standing	175	2.5	Rowing a boat 2.5 mph	300	4
Sweeping floor	100	1.5	Skiing 10 mph	600	8
Wringing by hand	265	3.5	Swimming 1/4 mile	300	4
			Table tennis	360	5
			Tennis	420	6
			Walking 2.5 mph	210	3
			Walking 3.5 mph	340	4.5

During an exercise program, if chest pain develops, the program must be stopped. Other symptoms of angina during exercise also need to be looked for. Pain in the elbow is a common symptom in healthy people playing tennis, but it can also indicate angina. One patient I know has anginal symptoms that begin with a bloating experience as soon as he starts to play tennis. He cured himself of this uncomfortable feeling by taking nitroglycerine under his tongue.

Conclusion: Exercise is contraindicated and dangerous to your life:

1. if you are having chest pain;
2. if the heart is abnormally enlarged;
3. if there is disease of the valve, such as aortic stenosis or idiopathic hypertrophic subaortic stenosis;
4. if your blood pressure is very elevated;
5. if there is a 60 percent closure of the left main coronary artery;

6. if you are over forty and have not had a stress test under a physician's supervision;
7. if you have just eaten or are tired;
8. or if the heart develops many irregular heartbeats during exercise.

Case: Mr. R.S. was a fifty-two-year-old man who developed angina for the first time. He smoked two packs of cigarettes a day, and his blood pressure was 160/100. His physician prescribed nitroglycerine, beta-blockers, and added calcium channel blockers. The patient started an exercise program after he was stress-tested. It was determined that he could safely reach a pulse rate of 120 beats per minute. He started his program by walking 2.5 miles an hour, gradually increasing it to 3.5 miles, which was equal to 4.5 mets or 240 calories per hour. As the weather got colder, he continued his walking exercise in the shopping mall. He slowly increased his physical activity and bought himself a stationary bicycle and set it at 5.5 mph, a speed at which he utilized 250 calories; he gradually increased it to 12 mph over the next year. His blood pressure dropped substantially, along with his weight. His angina disappeared entirely, and the physician slowly decreased his medications. Two years later, the patient was receiving only a long-acting beta-blocker, which he took in the morning and which maintained his pulse rate at 60. He is completely rehabilitated and it is unlikely that he will need coronary bypass surgery in the near future, his cholesterol having dropped to 150, and his HDL to 65.

What about Jogging?

Jim Fixx, the guru of jogging, was found dead lying on the side of the road. An autopsy revealed that he had advanced disease of three arteries. A forty-four-year-old director of

New York's Creedmore Hospital died while jogging along a Long Island road. A Health, Education, and Welfare analyst falls dead during a three-mile mass run in Washington to protest the HEW red tape. The head of the Miami Heart Institute collapses and dies while jogging at the age of forty-six. Sudden deaths occur throughout the United States during jogging that are not reported in the daily tabloids.

The majority of people who jog do not suffer, as a rule, any cardiac complications.

People of both sexes and all ages and sizes—sweating, groaning, faces flushed, wide-eyed—have rediscovered the ancient sport of running. Window displays are cluttered with proper running shoes and garments, and bookshelves are crowded with writings on the salutary effects of jogging, among which the best known is the book written by Jim Fixx. Many feel they have found the fountain of youth and longevity in a pair of sneakers and jogging shorts. Jogging has become the "in" thing for curing depressions and fatigue, increasing sexual abilities, and allegedly warding off a heart attack and prolonging life.

As we have seen, arteriosclerosis of the coronary arteries begins usually at an early age in our society, so by the time middle-aged individuals embark on their jogging, many have coronary arteries well on their way to becoming sclerotic and narrowed. Arteriosclerosis of the coronary arteries is a progressive illness which perhaps can be stopped with proper dieting, but so far there is no evidence that jogging reduces or prevents arteriosclerosis—or building up in the new blood vessels.

As a practicing cardiologist, I strongly advocate exercise and some jogging as a means of maintaining a fortified cardiovascular status. I strongly urge patients over the age of forty to have adequate testing to determine if arteriosclerosis has already started. This can be accomplished to some degree by thorough physical examination, a profile of the fat content of the blood—cholesterol, triglycerides, high-density lipoproteins—a resting electrocardiogram, and a cardiac stress test. Jogging is not a universal prescription. It needs to be assessed on an individual basis.

Persons with strong family histories of heart disease, who are obese, or who smoke cigarettes need to be carefully advised. I, for one, do not recommend jogging in a person over the age of forty if it leaves him or her like a washed-out rag. I find that one or two miles at a comfortable pace probably is not harmful. Jogging under the most strenuous conditions, as in the heart of winter, or when the weather is hot and humid, is dangerous.

I would like to emphasize again that jogging does not prevent a heart attack or sudden death, and it is not a substitute for a well-balanced emotional and physical life, and doesn't beat a fast-paced walk! A daily brisk, long walk (two to three miles) can be an excellent substitute for jogging!

III

CORONARY BYPASS SURGERY

7

Deciding on Bypass

Coronary bypass surgery is definitely indicated:

1. when the patient has angina, and there is evidence that the left main artery is more than 75 percent diseased (there is a 50 percent chance of dying in a year without the surgery);

2. when there is severe chest pain that is not improved with medical therapy;

3. when one, two, or three vessels have disease, i.e., are critically narrowed, and the quality of life is no longer acceptable to the patient because of chest pain; or

4. in the case of severe chest pain that does not improve after a heart attack or during a heart attack. In essence, it is the severity of the pain that will help determine whether surgery should be performed, along with how badly diseased the coronary arteries are and the state of function of the heart (ejection fraction).

Coronary bypass surgery may be avoided or delayed if there is moderate or minimal chest pain, even if there is involvement of one, two, or three blood vessels, especially if the heart function is good. In patients who have no symptoms and who are found to have abnormal arteries, surgery can be delayed indefinitely or until the time that pain appears. The Coronary Artery Surgery Study (CASS), conducted from 1975 to 1979, discovered that in patients who are suffering from mild to moderate angina and have good heart function, the annual death rate in surgically treated and medically treated patients is the same. Patients who have severe chest pain, or have disease of the left main artery (which occurs in approximately 5 to 10 percent of people studied), are, unfortunately, in a situation that dictates the need for surgery.

The Coronary Artery Surgery Study also discovered that surgical patients do have a better quality of life, since they require fewer medications, but the surgical groups did have more hospitalizations. The relief from angina, however, is the same in both groups. It should be pointed out that this study was performed at a time when we were not using channel calcium blockers, and it is possible that in the next study medically treated patients will fare even better than the surgical patients.

The Coronary Artery Surgery Study is recognized as the most complete study yet performed. Dr. Eugene Braunwald, a leading cardiologist from Boston, has also been advocating a conservative approach to the treatment of coronary artery disease ever since the first study, conducted by the Veterans Administration, of the treatment of patients with chronic angina. The results of this study were recorded in September, 1977, in the *New England Journal of Medicine.* Dr. Braunwald has been quoted as saying that bypass surgery may go the way of tonsillectomies—there will be a marked decrease in the number of operations.

At the present time, $4 billion is spent each year for this operation. The Coronary Artery Surgery Study estimated that 15 percent or more of operations could be delayed or perhaps avoided. This number means that a minimum of 25,000 patients could safely delay coronary bypass surgery and undergo medical treatment. This would save the nation

$625 million annually, calculated at an average cost per operation of $25,000. Undoubtedly, there are many gray areas involved, and the final decision concerning the operation should be an agreement between the informed patient and the physician. For example, there are times when only one artery, the left anterior descending artery, is severely diseased. Even though the patient has minimal symptoms, it might be advisable to operate, because this artery supplies a major portion of blood to the heart. There are numerous gray areas that have not been included in the Coronary Artery Bypass Study and that are still being studied.

In summary, the results of coronary bypass surgery in 1985 are generally good:

1. Ninety percent of the patients are freed of their angina;

2. the death rate is in the vicinity of 1.5 percent in uncomplicated cases; in patients over sixty-five, it is in the vicinity of 5 percent; and

3. the better the heart function is prior to surgery, the less possibility there is for complication and the greater the chances for survival.

However:

1. coronary bypass surgery does not prolong life, except in the case of left main artery disease, where the mortality rate is 50 percent per year. In mild or moderate angina, or asymptomatic patients, medical treatment is as good as surgical treatment and bypass surgery can be withheld, if the function of the heart is good;

2. bypass surgery can often be avoided if the patient is adequately medicated and follows a strict program of rehabilitation (weight reduction, low-cholesterol diet, cessation of smoking, exercise, and control of blood pressure);

3. patients who have surgery can expect a better quality of life, according to the studies, inasfar as less medications are given, but they can also expect more hospitalizations; and

4. bypass surgery alone does not prevent a subsequent heart attack. In an article published in the *Journal of the American College of Cardiology* (April 1984), it was concluded that progressive disease in the non-bypassed arteries and within bypass grafts is observed from five to twelve years after surgery. (It can be expected that the grafts will close at the rate of approximately 4 percent per year of all grafts, and by the end of ten years, 70 percent of the grafts will be closed and the patient may then have to again face the operation.)

According to the *Journal of Thoracic Cardiovascular Surgery* (March 1983), after three years the overall survival rate of bypass patients with an ejection fraction or target heart function below 20 percent was only 15 percent. However, ejection fractions above 25 percent had a survival rate of 60 percent at the end of three years. This study basically says that if the heart function is poor, the bypass patient has only a 15 percent chance of surviving more than three years. If the heart function is moderate, the survival rate can be 60 percent after three years.

Patients who have poor heart function, severe disease of the arteries, and moderate chest pain are advised surgery on an individual basis. Again, the quality of life is a major issue. All efforts certainly should be made to relieve severe pain, as long as the patient understands in full the increased risk that may be involved.

Patients who have minimal symptoms, and whose ejection fraction begins to deteriorate, as measured by a nuclear (MUGA) scan (from 50 percent to 35 percent, for example), are advised to have bypass surgery, or angioplasty if possible, to prevent further heart deterioration, even if they only have one vessel diseased.

As Dr. Richard Gorlin, chairman of the department of medicine at Mt. Sinai Hospital in New York City, so correctly and elegantly put it: "Vein grafts also have a relative morbidity or limited 'useful life' and are susceptible to the same disorders as the native coronary arteries in patients predisposed to arteriosclerosis."

Early closure of the graft is caused by thrombosis, while the late process is atherosclerotic. The best results from coronary bypass surgery can be expected in people who have good left-ventricular function and good distal vessels. The reason that the veins close off early is that there is a thickening of the wall *(fibrous intimal proliferation and fibrosis).* The current consensus is that patients who have a poor ejection fraction and minimal symptoms should also be advised to have surgery, even if only one or two blood vessels are diseased. Some patients may exhibit minimal pains and still have serious heart disease!

Case Histories

In the following section, I have related true case histories in order to specifically illustrate who needs bypass surgery. Not every situation is covered, but I have made every effort to describe the common situations when bypass surgery is or is not needed. For reasons not yet understood, the great majority of heart patients, up to 1985, have been males.

Case 1

- severe disease of the left main coronary artery—95 percent occlusion
- 95 percent occlusion also in the right coronary artery
- angina
- good ejection fraction

S.V., a forty-two-year-old warehouse manager who smoked two packs of cigarettes a day, suddenly developed a tightness in his chest while carrying packages to his truck. The pain lasted for ten minutes and then disappeared. Later

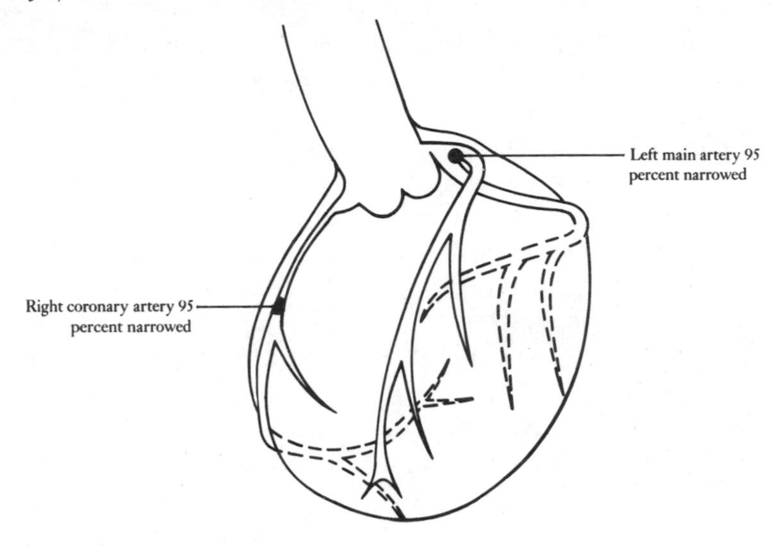

Figure 4. Case 1: Two-vessel disease

the same night, he had severe crunching pain over his breastbone, which spread down to his left arm, and he began to perspire profusely. His wife called the emergency number and the patient was very soon on his way to the local hospital. In the ambulance, an intravenous infusion was placed into his arm, and an electrocardiogram was taken. The blood pressure was 120/70 and the pulse was 100. This information was transmitted to the emergency room doctor.

At the hospital, the electrocardiogram did not show any changes that spelled a heart attack. The man received morphine for his pain and then was transferred to the coronary care unit. The pain did not reappear, the electrocardiogram did not change, and the heart enzymes remained normal. The doctors concluded that this patient had not had a heart attack, but that he had the classical symptoms of angina.

Before discharge from the hospital, an exercise stress test was performed. After his pulse rate reached 120, he complained of severe chest pain, and the electrocardiogram changed drastically. The S-T segment (which represents the electrical activity of the heart muscle) fell dangerously below the baseline, indicating a serious cardiac problem. The patient was returned to the coronary care unit and was observed for several more days, there still being no indication that he had suffered a heart attack.

The severe pain during the exercise stress test and the significantly abnormal electrocardiogram strongly suggested that the patient had serious disease of his coronary arteries. Three days later he was scheduled for cardiac catheterization, and in the meantime, nitroglycerine, beta-blockers, and channel-blocker medications were started. The patient remained in the hospital, still having chest pains that responded little to the treatment.

Cardiac catheterization disclosed that he had a left main artery that was 95 percent occluded and a right coronary artery that was 95 percent blocked, and circumflex artery stenosis of 75 percent. The ejection fraction was above 55 percent, which meant that his heart function remained good. Four days later, he underwent coronary bypass surgery with three vein grafts being placed, bypassing his obstructed arteries.

Comment: This forty-two-year-old man had severe disease involving his left main artery, including critical involvement of the right coronary artery. The unanimous decision to operate on this young man was based on numerous studies that concluded that patients who have the left main artery occluded have a 50 percent chance of dying in a year. The patient had a successful result. He gave up smoking and went on a strict reducing diet, has remained symptom-free for the past four years, and has been working ever since.

Case 2

- angina
- good ejection fraction

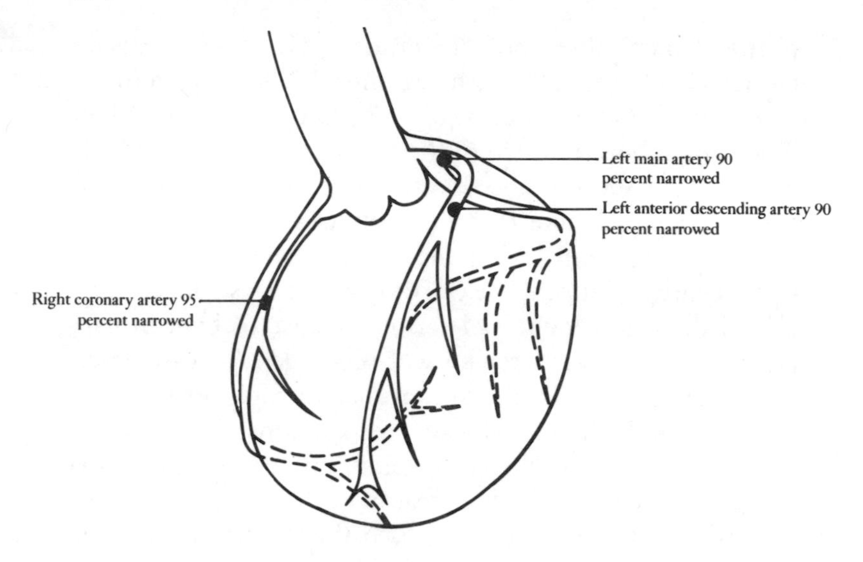

Figure 5. Case 2: Three-vessel disease

- 90 percent occlusion of left main artery
- 95 percent obstruction of right coronary artery
- 90 percent obstruction of left anterior descending artery
- three-vessel disease

A fifty-two-year-old man who smoked a pack of cigarettes every day complained of a nagging feeling in his chest of several days' duration, which he had noticed for the first time in the winter of 1980, while walking on the streets against the wind. His family history revealed that his father had had heart attacks, as well as diabetes.

The physician who examined him found his blood pressure to be 150/100, and the heart examination was normal. The electrocardiogram at rest was also within normal limits. The physician then advised a cardiac stress test. When the patient reached a pulse rate of 140, he began to complain of some dull feeling in his chest, and the stress test began to show 1.5 mm S-T segment changes. The test was discontinued and the pain disappeared. The physician felt that a thallium stress test should be added in order to have further evidence of the severity of the patient's coronary artery disease.

A thallium stress test verified the stress test findings. It showed that an area on the back and lateral side of the heart received inadequate amounts of blood. The patient also had a nuclear scan, which measured his heart function at 57 percent. He received nitroglycerine and a beta-blocker, which reduced his pulse rate to 55. The patient's pain disappeared and he had a sense of well-being for a period of two weeks. However, he continued to smoke in spite of his doctor's admonitions. Then his pain reappeared, and the doctor increased the medications. Once again the pain subsided. The patient continued to do well for the next four weeks, but then the chest pain surfaced again with greater intensity, in spite of maximum dosages of his beta-blockers.

Cardiac catheterization was performed and disclosed that he had a left main artery that was 90 percent occluded, a right coronary artery with a 95 percent obstruction, and a 90 percent obstruction of the left anterior descending artery. The patient underwent coronary bypass surgery of four blood vessels.

Comment: There was a unanimous decision that this patient should have bypass surgery because the disease of his three arteries was far advanced. Also, because of his main artery's being occluded by more than 75 percent, his chance of dying was great. The patient had successful results, with complete disappearance of his pain, and he was returned to his work.

Case 3

- angina not relieved by medications
- good heart function
- two diseased blood vessels—90 percent occlusion

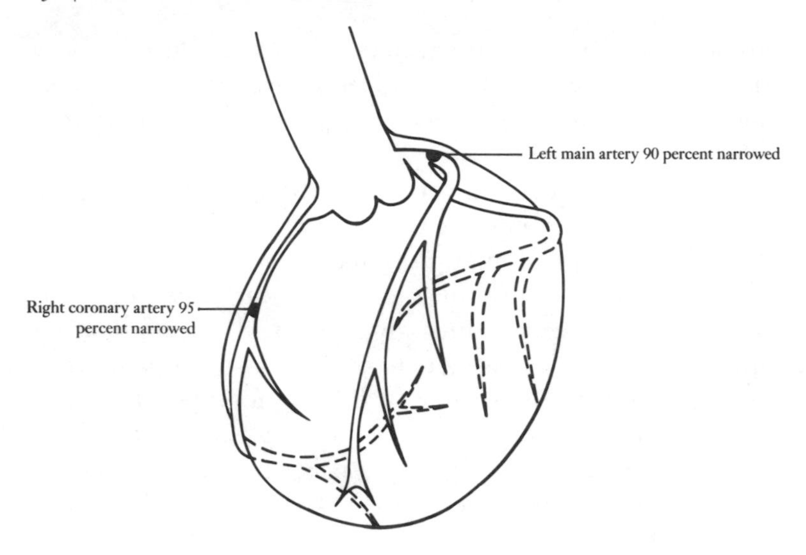

Figure 6. Case 3: Two-vessel disease

A fifty-nine-year-old businessman, one morning, while raising his garage door, complained of excruciating pain in his chest. He recalls that "the pain felt as if an elephant was sitting on my chest, and I could barely breathe; the sweat was pouring down."

He was dispatched to the emergency room of his local hospital. An electrocardiogram disclosed that he had suffered a heart attack. He was placed into the coronary care unit, and after twenty-four hours his pain disappeared. From the course of his hospital stay, it appeared as if he had suffered an uncomplicated heart attack, and on the tenth day, he was discharged with medications: nitroglycerine and beta-blockers. Several weeks later, his pain reappeared with great intensity while he was lying quietly in bed. He was readmitted into the hospital, but this time he was found not to have had a heart attack. It was learned later from his physician that he had been under a great deal of business pressure. His job was threatened and his relationship with his wife had deteriorated after twenty-three years of marriage. After discharge, the medication was increased, but he continued having some degree of pain each day, varying from mild to severe, which was promptly relieved with nitroglycerine tablets.

The patient underwent cardiac catheterization, which disclosed that he had two blood vessels that were 90 percent diseased, the right coronary artery and the left anterior descending artery. A cardiologist informed him that he had approximately a 2 percent chance of dying in a year. His heart function was normal (the ejection fraction was 58 percent); however, he continued to have chest pain and he found his life was not acceptable. He underwent triple bypass surgery, but the pain reappeared in several months.

Comment: The surgery was necessary because of the severity of the pain that was not relieved medically. It was only temporarily successful because nothing changed in the patient's life, neither his personal habits nor the easing of his tensions.

These cases represent probably a unanimous opinion among cardiologists about candidates who should have bypass surgery. All the patients had good function of the left ventricle as measured by the ejection fraction, and therefore had less risk during the operation. The better the function of the left ventricle at the time of operation, the less chance there is of dying. The mortality rate of the operation should not be more than 1 to 2 percent. If the left ventricular function, or the ejection fraction, as measured by the MUGA, or during cardiac catheterization, is in the vicinity of 25 percent, the mortality rate rises sharply to 5 to 6 percent.

Case 4

- left anterior descending artery 75 percent occluded
- right coronary artery 90 percent occluded

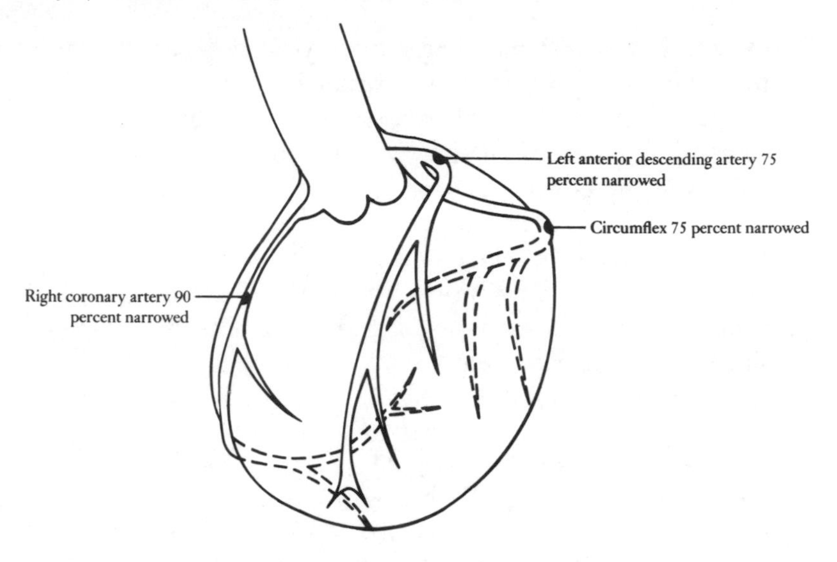

Figure 7. Case 4: Three-vessel disease

- circumflex 75 percent occluded
- good ejection fraction
- angina

A fifty-nine-year-old man, highly compulsive by nature, knew he was suffering from angina, but he did not seek any medical attention. Each morning, when he arrived at the office, he had pains in his chest that lasted for five to ten minutes as he sat at his desk planning his day's activity. He relieved them by taking a warm glass of water, and finally, because of the urging of his wife, he went to see his physician. He told his physician: "I think I'm suffering from angina, and I would like you to prescribe medication for me."

The physician listened carefully to the history of pressure and tightness in the front of his chest, which sometimes went up to his neck or down to his arm, not accompanied by any perspiration, but rather with a feeling of weakness, which, a few minutes later, was relieved spontaneously. The examination of the man disclosed that he had a blood pressure of 180/110. The electrocardiogram was normal, his cholesterol was 320, his HDL was 22, and his LDL was elevated. The man felt that the symptoms did not in any way interfere with his life, but that they were just a nuisance to him. They had never become severe enough to prevent him from going to work or to stop him from what he was doing.

A cardiac stress test was performed, which, as predicted, showed an abnormality when the patient reached a pulse of 150, with 2-mm S-T segment depression. The patient was reluctant to tell the physician that he was having pain. He decided that he wanted to know the state of his arteries and insisted that he have a cardiac catheterization even before medication was tried.

A cardiac catheterization disclosed that his left anterior descending artery was closed by 75 percent, the right coronary artery by 90 percent, and the circumflex by 75 percent. The left main artery, however, was free of disease. It was furthermore determined that the ejection fraction of the heart was 60 percent. The man had read of a study, called the European Cooperative Study, which investigators from twelve European countries participated in between the years 1973 and 1976 and reported in 1977. It was reported in this study that of those patients who had bypass surgery, 95 percent were alive at the end of two years, compared to 89 percent of those treated medically. He felt that this study was significant and decided to undergo bypass surgery. The operation was successful and he was symptom-free.

Comment: In an American Veterans Administration study of July 1981, patients with three-vessel disease were shown to do better with surgery than with medical treatment, and this was the consensus until 1983. Our decision to advise surgery at that time was based on the studies. Today, since the CASS (Coronary Artery Surgical Study) reported in 1983, many cardiologists feel that with three-vessel disease, good ejection fraction, and minimal symptoms, patients could hold off on having surgery until the time they do become more symptomatic or their heart deteriorates.

Case 5

- three diseased vessels
- good heart function
- left anterior descending artery 85 percent narrowed
- right coronary artery 75 percent narrowed
- circumflex artery 50 percent narrowed

Bill was in his mid-fifties when he developed angina, and he was set in his mind that he wanted "something really done about his coronary arteries." He was arrogant, a heavy smoker, and suffered from mild hypertension. His cardiac catheterization revealed his left main artery was free of disease. His left anterior descending artery was 85 percent

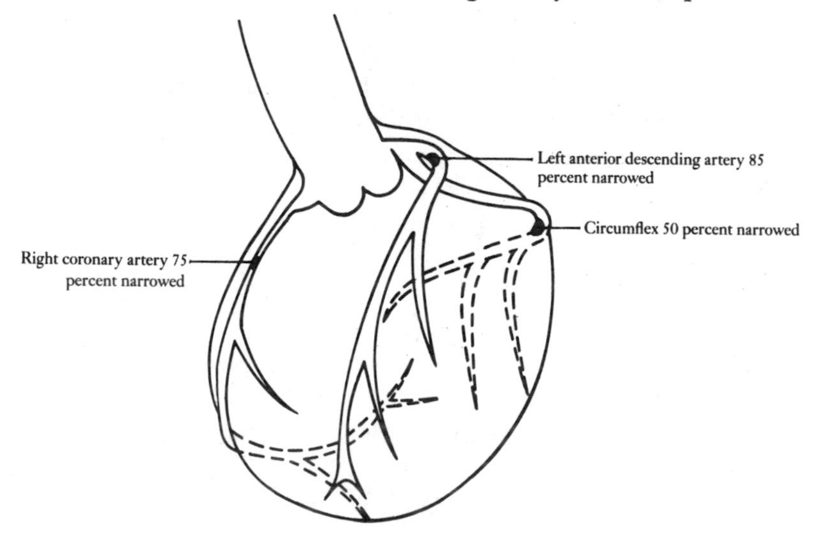

Figure 8. Case 5: Three-vessel disease

stenosed, the right 75 percent, and the circumflex 50 percent. He did not want to take any medications and he did have successful results from the surgery.

Comment: Although Bill would have had the same results with medical treatment, he did not want to bother with medications. The doctor did explain to him that the operation was not a permanent cure, and that in seven years he had a 50 percent chance of the grafts closing and he might need another operation.

Case 6

- heart attack
- shock
- emergency surgery for three critically diseased coronary arteries

A sixty-two-year-old printer suffered with angina for many years until beta-blockers arrived and he became symp-

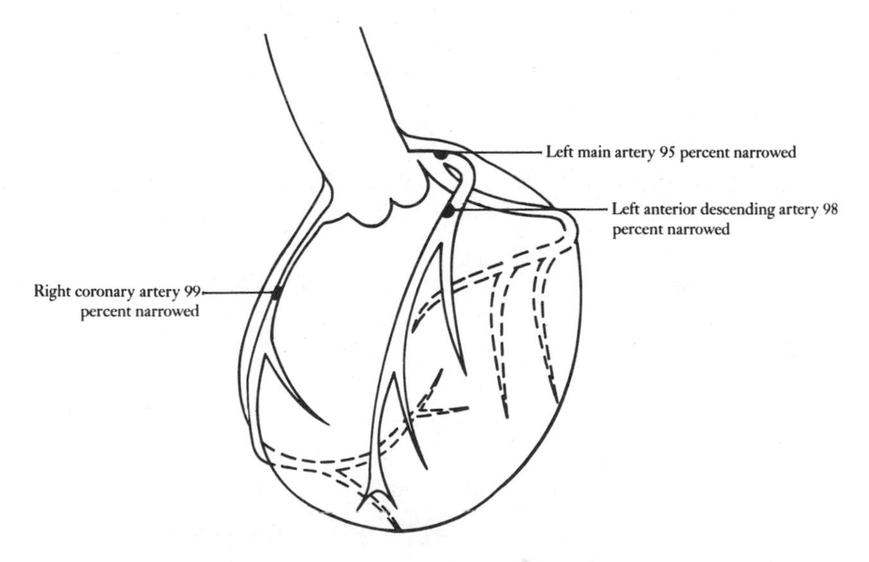

Figure 9. Case 6: Three-vessel disease

tom-free. One Christmas morning his chest pain reappeared and was not relieved by the nitroglycerine he placed under his tongue. When the pain continued for nearly half an hour, his wife rushed him to the local hospital, where the electrocardiogram demonstrated an anterior wall infarction. He continued to have chest pain in spite of receiving I.V. nitroglycerine and beta-blockers. His blood pressure dropped, his pain increased, and it was evident that the printer was passing into cardiac shock.

A device called the *balloon pump* was inserted to take over the work of the heart and perfuse the coronary arteries. The intra-aortic balloon pump is inserted through an artery into the leg and increases the flow of blood through the coronary arteries. It also reduces the amount of work the heart has to do and gives the surgeon some extra time to prepare for bypass surgery, if the surgery is feasible.

Balloon pumping, a form of taking over the work of the heart, has been used for more than ten years. The balloon, inserted in the aorta, is inflated by compressed air from a pump and forces the blood into the coronary arteries while the heart is relaxing. When the heart again contracts, the balloon is automatically deflated. Inflation and deflation of the balloon are in rhythm with the patient's heart rate.

The patient underwent cardiac catheterization, which disclosed that all his three coronary arteries were critical, obstructed. Emergency bypass surgery was performed, and he received four grafts to his heart. Several weeks later, he was home, his life having been saved by the operation. Emergency bypass surgery is risky, but sometimes, as in this example, the patient would succumb if he did not have the surgery.

Case 7

- large segment occluded—95 percent—of the left anterior descending artery

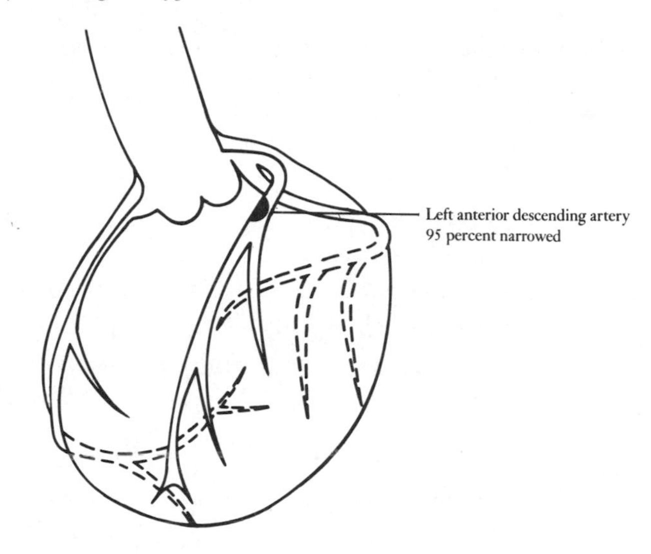

Figure 10. Case 7: One-vessel disease

- good ejection fraction
- mild angina

A thirty-five-year-old business executive developed mild chest pain while he was jogging. His father had died of heart disease at forty-five, and his brother had sustained a myocardial infarction at the age of thirty-two. The examination of his heart was normal and his blood pressure read 110/70, but the stress and thallium stress disclosed a large defect in his heart. His cholesterol was 280, the triglycerides were 220, and the HDL was 25. Cardiac catheterization disclosed a large segment of the left anterior descending artery to be occluded by 95 percent. In this case, this artery was the main supplier of most of the front of the heart. Because he had such a tight closure of his artery, he underwent bypass surgery, using the internal mammary artery.

Comment: Because of the severity of his arterial involvement, although it involved only one artery, this young patient fell outside the average type of patient who could wait for bypass surgery. With his significant family history, the decision was unanimous to perform the operation.

Case 8

- left anterior descending artery occluded by 75 percent
- no symptoms

L.A., a forty-four-year-old executive, went for his annual physical. He was 5′8″ and weighed 190 pounds. His blood pressure was found to be 160/100. His electrocardiogram was entirely normal. As part of the annual physical, he had a lipid profile, which included a serum cholesterol of 320, an HDL of 30, and an elevated LDL. He also had a treadmill test performed as part of his physical. He reached a maximum pulse rate of 185 with no symptoms, but the electrocardiogram showed a 2-mm S-T segment depression. The examining doctor showed great concern seeing the abnormal

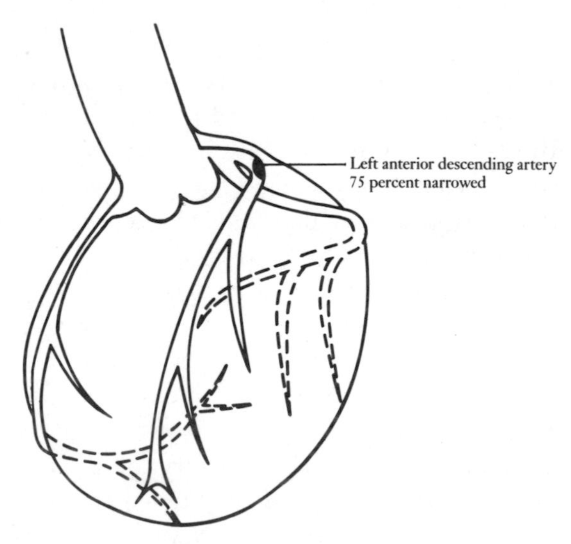

Figure 11. Case 8: One-vessel disease

stress test and advised cardiac catheterization. Prior to undergoing the catheterization, a thallium stress test was done, which showed a moderate defect on the front of the heart. A nuclear scan disclosed an ejection fraction of 75 percent, a good reading.

Cardiac catheterization was performed at the hospital, demonstrating that the left anterior descending artery was 75 percent occluded. The patient was advised to give up cigarette smoking and to follow both a very strict reducing diet, with a cholesterol intake of less than 300 mg per day, and a low-salt diet. Surgery was not advised, since the doctor's judgment, supported by recent studies, was that the medical treatment in this case was as promising as the surgical treatment. If symptoms did develop angioplasty or an operation could later be considered.

Comment: The patient stopped smoking, lost weight, and his blood pressure came under control with beat-blockers. He continues to remain free of symptoms.

Numerous studies support this medical decision. The Seattle Heart Watch measured the effect on survival of medical treatment for 277 patients and surgical treatment for 392 patients. These people, like our patient, had no symptoms and had one major artery blocked by 70 percent. The report of this study, issued in 1980, showed that patients with one-vessel disease and good ejection fraction did just as well with medical treatment, and that prophylactic bypass surgery did not significantly improve long-term survival. Similar findings were confirmed by a Veterans Administration study in 1977.

In the most recent study of the coronary artery surgery randomized trial (CASS), it was discovered that the annual mortality rate for single-vessel disease was 1.1 percent of patients treated medically, compared to 0.8 percent of patients treated surgically, which is not statistically significant.

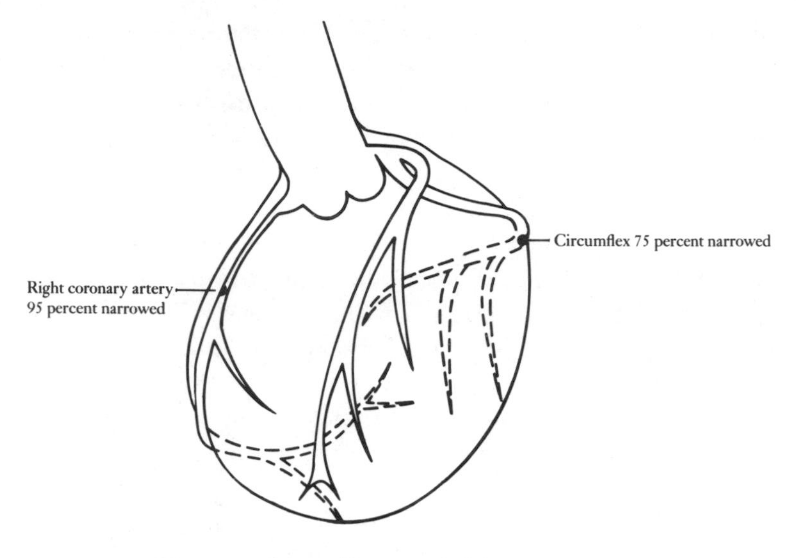

Figure 12. Case 9: Two-vessel disease

Case 9

- heart attack
- right coronary artery closed by 95 percent
- circumflex artery closed by 75 percent
- good ejection fraction
- two-vessel disease

A fifty-four year-old physician suffered a heart attack while he was working in his office. Before discharge from the hospital, a cardiac stress test recorded abnormal changes of 1.5 mm, with no chest pain. The heart attack had involved the inferior wall of the heart, and he decided to undergo cardiac catheterization, which disclosed his right coronary artery was closed by 95 percent and the circumflex artery by 75 percent. There was a good ejection fraction. The doctor did not have bypass surgery.

Comment: He reduced his work schedule, took on a partner, spent more time with his family, and started on an exercise and dietary program. He has remained symptom-free for the past three years. The doctor did not have to have bypass surgery, because his death risk would be the same whether or not he had the operation. The yearly death rate with two-vessel disease, and good heart function, according to the latest coronary artery bypass surgery statistics, is approximately 1.6 percent, and as long as the doctor remained symptom-free, there was no need to operate on him at the time.

Case 10

- angina not controlled with adequate dosage
- right coronary artery 100 blocked
- left anterior descending 75 narrowed
- two-vessel disease

George is a sixty-one-year-old active male who suffered from high cholesterol all his life. His family history revealed

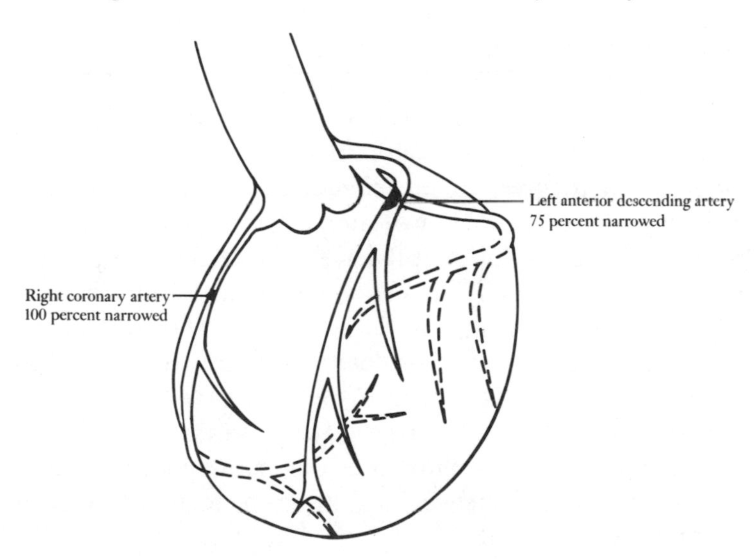

Figure 13. Case 10: Two-vessel disease

that an older brother and his father had had heart attacks. He made no attempt at dietary control or to stop smoking. He had a long history of poorly controlled hypertension. His doctor told him that with a blood pressure of 165/110 and a cholesterol level of 310, according to the coronary risk handbook made available by the American Heart Association he had a 30 percent probability of developing a heart attack within a six-year period. (If the blood pressure was 120/80, and the serum cholesterol was 185, there would have been a 4.6 percent probability.) This man finally did sustain a heart attack. Months later, he had periodic episodes of mild angina when walking uphill. He did not lose weight, and his blood pressure was not controlled because he took the medication inconsistently. He received beta-blockers, but the dosage was inadequate since the pulse rate remained around 85 and his blood pressure remained at 180/110. Cardiac catheterization demonstrated that the right coronary artery was 100 percent blocked and the left anterior descending was 75 percent narrowed. He was considered a treatment failure and was advised to have bypass surgery.

George had read that second opinions are a good idea. The doctor who rendered the second opinion felt George had not received an adequate trial of treatment. He convinced him to give up his cigarettes and go on a strict reducing diet. His cholesterol intake was lowered to 200 mg per day, his beta-blocker pills were increased to drop his pulse rate to 60, and he was encouraged to increase his physical activity progressively. At the end of several months, the pain had completely disappeared, his blood pressure was controlled, and his weight gain began to decrease. George had not felt so good in years.

Comment: This case illustrates that sometimes treatment failures may be primarily caused by an inadequate dosage of beta-blockers.

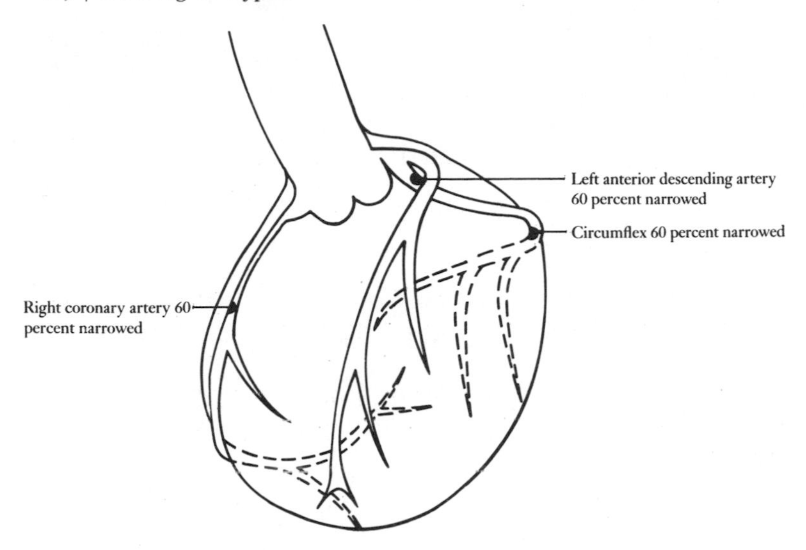

Figure 14. Case 11: Three-vessel disease

Case 11

- no symptoms
- three vessels narrowed by 60 percent
- good ejection fraction

S.J., an obese, fifty-five-year-old, non-athletic truckdriver, a heavy smoker, was required to have an annual physical examination in order to renew his license. The examination disclosed that his blood pressure was 220/110, which was markedly elevated, and his pulse was 75. The lung examination showed early emphysema, and the heart examination was normal. An electrocardiogram showed evidence of an old heart attack. The patient did not have any chest pain. He had only a moderate cough. The physician advised him to have cardiac catheterization to decide how much damage to coronary arteries there was and to confirm that he had indeed had a heart attack.

Comment: In this case, a cardiac catheterization certainly was not necessary, but it did disclose that he had three vessels that were diseased by 60 percent and a heart function that was over 65 percent. The doctor felt that he should have bypass surgery performed. In this case, not only was the cardiac catheterization not needed, but it was also certainly not necessary for him to have bypass surgery. He did seek a second opinion, and was advised to undergo a strict rehabilitation program, including beta-blockers, and not to undergo surgery.

With the new medication, channel calcium blockers, we now have an extra tool to keep patients symptom-free. When there is two-vessel involvement, the medical treatment is as good as the surgical treatment, and surgery probably does not prolong life. At a later date, surgery may be necessary if symptoms develop or the heart function begins to deteriorate.

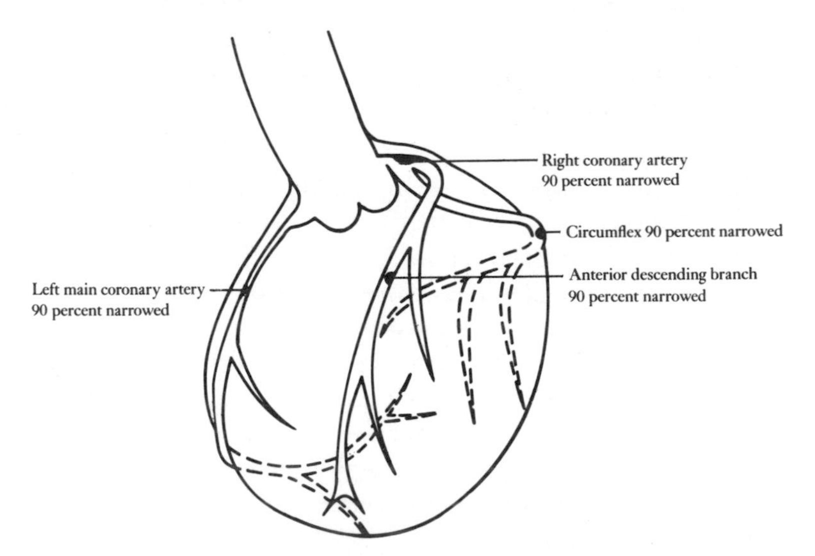

Figure 15. The ideal candidate for surgery: vessels occluded; severe angina; good heart function; good terminal vessels to attach graft

Case 12

- typical angina but no arteriosclerosis of the coronary arteries

Marvin, forty-nine, was an extraordinarily high-strung person "from the day he was born." His mother recalls how he wiggled in his crib and never sat still for a second. Even as a young man he spoke in an explosive tone and his hands were moist; his heart was always racing. Things only got worse as he got older, except that whereas previously he had complained of stomach pains, which were coming from an ulcer, and migraine headaches, and multiple allergies, he now complained of chest pain. The chest pain was classical angina in character, and the only difference was that it occurred while he was sitting quietly. At night, he told the doctor, he heard his heart racing and the pain would start.

During one of his episodes of chest pain, which happened while he was sitting on the examining table, the alert physician quickly took an electrocardiogram. The famous S-T segment on the electrocardiogram suddenly became elevated, and the doctor had his diagnosis. Since the patient was a young person, and had been complaining of continual chest pain for years, the doctor feared that perhaps his illness was much more severe than it had first seemed to be.

At cardiac catheterization, the coronary arteries were entirely normal; however, there was evidence that they were twitching and going into spasm. The treatment prescribed consisted of nitroglycerine and a channel calcium blocker, and it was successful.

Comment: The patient did not need bypass surgery, and as a matter of fact, if bypass surgery had been performed, he might still have had chest pain from spasms of the arteries that were not grafted.

As discussed in an earlier chapter, coronary artery spasm

is now a well-known condition. It can be an illness by itself without any evidence of atherosclerosis of the arteries, or it may be associated with clogged arteries. It is believed by many cardiologists that coronary artery spasm is an important component of angina and should be considered in every person whose angina occurs at rest. In patients who have blockage of the artery, superimposed coronary artery spasms can cause a heart attack, sometimes fatal. (A leading investigator of coronary artery spasm, as noted earlier, is Dr. Artilio Massari, who elegantly demonstrated the condition as an important portion of the symptomatology of coronary artery disease. During the attack of spasms, the coronary arteries become narrowed, which then impedes the flow of blood.)

Dr. M. Prinzmetal, in 1959, described patients with angina occurring at rest, accompanied by the S-T segment elevation. This condition is now known as *Prinzmetal angina.*

The calcium channel blockers, or calcium antagonists, are effective in blocking the spasms. Calcium channel blocker medications should be added in patients whose angina does not respond to nitroglycerine and beta-blockers, because spasms may be an important component of their illness.

The complete medical treatment of angina today includes nitroglycerine, beta-blockers, and the addition of the calcium channel blockers, especially if angina takes place at rest or has not been relieved by conventional treatment, including weight reduction, blood pressure control, cessation of smoking, and an exercise program. Patients with mild angina should not be sent to surgery as medical failures unless a complete treatment has been prescribed.

Previous epidemiological studies have not included patients who have been receiving calcium channel blockers. The medically treated patients might have done even better.

Case 13

- angina caused by coronary artery spasm

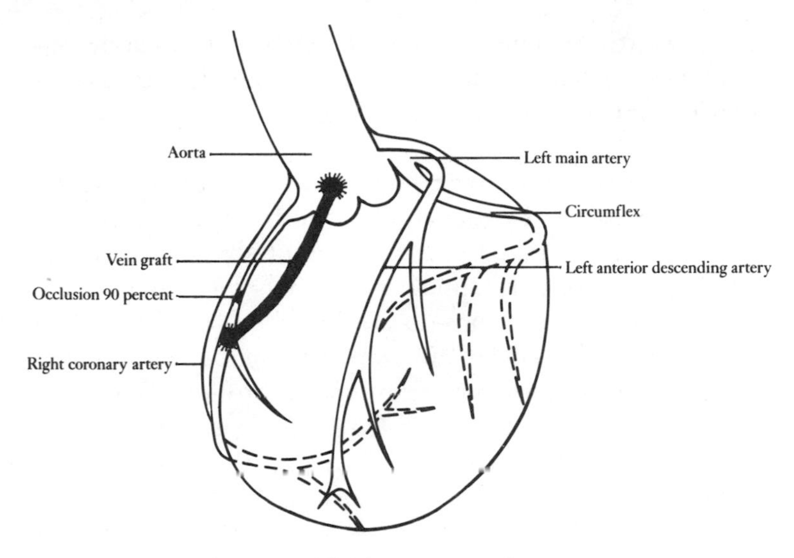

Figure 16. The bypass operation

A sixty-two-year-old man developed classical symptoms of coronary artery disease. His chest pain was present upon exertion, and also when he was resting quietly in bed. It became clear from his stress test and thallium stress test that there was evidence of moderate to severe coronary artery disease. Nitroglycerine and beta-blockers were prescribed, but the patient continued to have chest pain whenever he became aggravated, or when he was simply sitting quietly at home. Watching television or an exciting movie caused him to have chest pain, which was promptly relieved with nitroglycerine. Sexual intercourse, however, did not cause chest pain.

In 1980, when he heard of Dr. Maseri's work on channel blockers and coronary artery spasm, he volunteered to enter a research project. Calcium channel blockers were added to his treatment, and his angina disappeared.

Comment: Although it was never documented by cardiac catheterization that he had coronary artery spasm, his story was suggestive enough for his cardiologist to include calcium channel blockers in his treatment. He remains symptom-free and carries on an active life.

The elderly patient, over sixty-five, is considered a high-risk individual for bypass surgery. For that matter, almost any surgery performed over the age of sixty-five is risky. Organs, unfortunately, simply do not work as well as when one is younger. The lungs do not breathe as well, the brain does not have the same circulation as a twenty-year-old, and so on. The elderly patient's risk of dying from the operation has been reported as anywhere from 0 to 21 percent, whereas the mortality rate from bypass surgery for those under sixty-five is in the vicinity of 1 to 2 percent. Complications are more severe, particularly those involving the nervous system. In addition, the risk of complications from cardiac catheterization and angiography is greater. The hospital stay tends to be longer for older patients. Older people also tend to have more severe disease of the coronary arteries. Left main coronary artery disease, which has a 5 percent or so incidence in people who are younger, has an incidence of 15 percent in people who are older. The overall mortality rate of people over the age of sixty-five was 5.2 percent of the 1,086 patients studied, as compared to 1.9 percent in those who were under sixty-five.

Coronary bypass surgery should thus be avoided whenever possible in patients who are over sixty-five, since the prognosis is much more guarded. Again, if the left main artery is diseased and the patient has three-vessel disease with moderate symptoms, then surgery should not be withheld. Undoubtedly, even if the patient is seventy or older, if he has severe angina which is not responding to treatment and the quality of life is poor, surgery should be performed, but only after a vigorous attempt has been made with medication.

"He is too old to be operated on" is not true, either. Older patients have just as much right to be free of symptoms, and every medical effort should of course be made; surgery should certainly be performed if there is no other alternative.

Performing bypass surgery on arteries that are diseased but that do not cause any symptoms is not today considered necessary. Statistics have shown that in people who have no symptoms, the death rate per year is the same whether surgery is or is not performed. Prophylactic bypass surgery should not be done.

The above cases serve to illustrate a few of the conditions that determine if bypass surgery is needed or not. There are many times when the pathology is much more complicated than I have illustrated, and of course each case is unique. For example, two-vessel symptomatic disease should be operated on if it involves a 90 percent lesion of the left anterior descending artery and a 90 percent proximal lesion of the circumflex artery, which is equivalent to three vessels diseased, as these two vessels supply most of the heart.

8

The Heart Operation

AT the start of World War I, some heart surgery was being performed, but surgeons were reluctant to operate because as soon as the chest was opened, the lungs collapsed. During World War II, there were a few cases of retained missiles (bullets, shell fragments) that were removed from the walls of the heart. One of the major problems in developing open-heart surgery was to develop a pump to take over the work of the heart. The heart has to be paralyzed in order for the surgeon to repair the abnormalities. Numerous researchers designed different heart pumps, and finally, in 1951, Dr. Clarence Dennis, of the University of Minnesota, used a pump designed by Dr. John Gibson, of Philadelphia, and fixed a hole in the heart of a six-year-old child.

Dr. Claude Beck, in 1932, was concerned that there were some hearts "too young to die." He hypothesized that if there was a way of getting a blood supply into the heart muscle, an operation could be created whereby new arteries grow into the heart, thereby possibly curing angina. In February of 1935, Dr. Beck did operate and made a hole in the healthy sac that covers the heart (the pericardium) and placed talc into the sac to stimulate an inflammation. As new tissue grew from the sac, a new blood supply also developed into the heart. Seven months later, the patient no longer had chest pain. He reasoned that the covering of the heart had grown new arteries into the heart. The inflammation had stimulated growth of new blood vessels.

Different types of operations were designed to help patients suffering from angina. One kind of operation was performed to cut the nerve supply *(sympathectomy)*, another to remove the outer layers of the heart, which Dr. Dwight Harkin of Boston performed. The first surgeon to actually put new blood channels into the heart was Dr. Arthur Vineberg, a remarkable scientist and surgeon who taught anatomy before World War II. He was convinced that the two arteries that lie beneath the breastbone (the internal mammary arteries) could be separated and implanted in the heart. He first started experimenting with animals, with great success, and in 1950, he performed his first implant into the left wall of the heart, creating a new channel, bypassing the narrowed coronary arteries. From the implanted artery, some vessels did grow to the surrounding tissue. It was known throughout the world as the *Vineberg operation.* But this still was not the solution. Dr. Vineberg was unable to persuade the medical world until angiography showed that a communication could be established between an implanted artery and the coronary circulation.

It was Dr. Sones' demonstration of the coronary arteries in 1958 that prompted Dr. Michael DeBakey of Houston to attempt coronary bypass surgery. The patient died and Dr. DeBakey did not follow up at that time. It was Drs. René Favalaro and D. Effler, from the Cleveland Clinic, who first used a vein from a leg to bypass an obstruction.

The idea is simple enough. The *saphenous* is *vein* removed from the leg and attached on one end to a small opening made in the aorta; the other end is attached below the blockage in the coronary artery. The blood now flows from the aorta, bypasses the obstruction, and moves through the saphenous vein (or the internal mammary artery), beyond the obstruction. Physicians throughout the country challenged the concept and were a long time in accepting that coronary bypass surgery is a brilliant achievement in medicine. Patients who used to suffer for years with the scary and painful anginal symptoms now could live normal lives again.

When bypass surgery first came on the scene some fifteen years ago, skeptics abounded. An experiment, which was valid, was tried by Dr. E. Grey Dimond, a renowned cardiologist in Kansas. He questioned the operation to the extent that he convinced surgeons to perform a sham operation to see whether the patient would get better regardless of the procedure. The sham operation consisted of making a mere skin incision on the chest. There was improvement in most patients regardless of whether they received the actual or the sham operation. Dr. Dimond noted that 32 percent with severe coronary artery disease were improved. Those patients who were not operated on but only had the skin incision had a 43 percent improvement. Although it was a small, limited study, Dr. Dimond felt it was statistically significant that both categories of patients were markedly improved. He concluded that the operation was successful because of psychological reasons—the placebo effect.

Chemical agents have been used throughout history, and generally this form of treatment has not been harmful. Countless herbs and potions, and the wearing of bracelets, amulets, and rings, all have helped to relieve pain. Placebo effects can actually result in physical changes. In one experiment, patients were told that they were receiving a drug that narrowed their pupils. Seven of the fifteen patients developed narrowed pupils, even though they were receiving a sugar pill. Patients have also reported side effects from only sugar pills—headaches, sleepiness, nausea, dizzy spells, palpitations, and so forth. Some patients have even become addicted to a placebo. This is why careful, controlled studies need to be conducted, because physicians realize that treatment must be scientifically evaluated, since there is always the possibility of the placebo effect in obtaining symptomatic relief.

The coronary bypass operation, however, is certainly not a placebo. Oxygenated blood is brought from the great vessels, through the graft, into the coronary artery and then to the oxygen-starving heart muscle. Any of the coronary arteries can be bypassed—the left, the right, the circumflex—providing there are normal vessels, or near-normal vessels, to which to make the hookups. If the vessel below the obstruction is very narrow, correction may not be possible.

Angina is eliminated or improved in 80 to 90 percent of patients. There is an expected 20 percent failure rate resulting from the surgery, which means the angina has not improved, or has even worsened. The reappearance of angina results from the graft's becoming occluded.

There is now a resurgence in the use of the internal mammary artery rather than the saphenous vein from the legs. The mammary artery has a much longer period of remaining open. It becomes less clogged, and for some reason, it is not affected by arteriosclerosis to the same degree as the other arteries. Every person has two mammary arteries, a right and a left, on either side of the breastbone. The mammary artery is sometimes too small to be placed into a large coronary artery. If the heart is markedly thickened, it may not be appropriate to use such a small artery, since the smaller the channel, the less blood arrives. If more than one coronary artery needs to be replaced, one of the mammary arteries can be used for one replacement and the saphenous vein(s) of the legs for the other(s). It is technically more difficult to place a mammary artery than a vein, requiring special training and experience.

An additional advantage of the mammary artery is that it can be connected directly, whereas the vein has to be bent.

The mammary artery also much more closely approximates the opening of the native coronary artery. An incision obviously does not have to be made in the leg to remove the vein, which results in prolonged discomfort. (Indeed, some patients complain that the leg pain is the worst part of the operation.)

The mammary artery is, in the long run, superior to the veins. It takes a little longer to suture, and in emergency bypass surgery, the surgeon uses the leg vein because surgery can be performed much more swiftly.

At the American Heart Association's 56th Scientific Session (1983), the surgeons at the Cleveland Clinic discovered that 90 percent of the internal mammary artery remained open after five to twelve years, in contrast to 55 percent of those who had the vein grafts.

Choosing a Surgeon

Today, choosing a surgeon for heart surgery is not difficult. A thoracic and cardiac surgeon is someone who has spent at least two additional years of specialized training in surgery of the heart and lungs. (After completing medical school, a general surgeon has completed at least five years of specialized training in an accredited surgical residency program.)

It is perfectly reasonable for a patient to ask a physician about his qualifications. As a general rule, it is best to select a heart surgeon who has been board certified by the American Board of Surgery and the American Board of Thoracic Surgery. If he is a Fellow of the American College of Surgeons, this reflects that much more credit. A surgeon so certified has been approved to have a high level of judgment and requisite skill, but a surgeon not certified can still, to be sure, be superb. The patient can obtain this information from the *Directory of Medical Specialties* and the *American*

Medical Directory, which are available in all public libraries. In the *Directory,* information can be obtained regarding the doctor's age, his education, training, and the societies to which he belongs. By calling the local medical school or the chapter of the American Heart Association, similar information can be found. It is the consensus of the National Heart, Lung and Blood Institute, published in the *Federal Register,* that a heart surgeon should perform a minimum of three operations per week in order to keep his skills intact.

The hospital in which you are going to be operated on is just as important as the surgeon you select. It should have updated facilities, a well-trained nursing staff, and a record of excellence, and the number of heart operations performed each year should, at the least, exceed two hundred.

The patient should feel free to ask the surgeon specific questions regarding alternatives, risks, complications, and benefits. Further, it is appropriate to ask the surgeon how many times he has performed this operation, and to ask him to explain the procedure.

Being an advocate of second opinion, I recommend that if there is any doubt at all in the patient's mind, a second opinion should be sought. A second opinion is especially necessary when the patient complains of minimal symptoms (or has no symptoms at all) and is yet advised to have surgery when medical treatment has not been tried. Older patients, in particular, who have a higher risk rate and may have poor function of the heart, should get a second opinion if the symptoms are minimal. Because a patient has had a heart attack does not necessarily mean that he should have bypass surgery. Some surgeons and cardiologists advocate that bypass surgery should be performed in order to prevent another attack—a disputable position.

On the day you arrive at the hospital, bring the list of medications you are taking, and do not stop any of them unless advised to do so by your doctor. Even if you are taking "only" aspirins, be sure to tell the doctor.

The routine of the hospital the day before surgery may differ in different hospitals. In teaching hospitals, for example, medical students, interns, residents, and student nurses will come to interview and examine the patient. Your history will be reviewed and discussed, either at the bedside or within hearing distance. This is part of the training program of a university hospital and it is essential; future operations could not be performed without this training. The patient should realize that many of the things that are said do not refer to him directly. If at any time the patient feels that he is being over-examined, he has the right to refuse such examining, and if at any time he has questions or feels that he heard something he is unhappy about, he should quickly ask what was meant. There are nurses, medical students, and doctors around the ward to ask what is meant. If you are afraid or embarrassed to ask the questions, a spouse or friend can help.

Sometime before the operation, the patient will be asked to sign a consent form, a legal document that gives the surgeon permission to operate. The patient is again made aware of the benefits and the risks of the surgery. This is another good time for the patient and family to ask questions. As a wise man once said: "It is not questions that are ever foolish, only the answers."

Patients' Bill of Rights

Most hospitals have a booklet available to patients, stipulating their rights in the hospital—rights pertaining to choices of treatment.

The following is excerpted from an American Hospital Association statement:

1. The patient has the right to appropriate, considerate,

and courteous care, regardless of the source of payment for his care.

2. The patient, or an appropriate person acting in his behalf, has a right to receive from his physician complete information regarding his diagnosis, treatment, and prognosis in terms he can understand. He has the right to know by name the physician responsible for directing his care.

3. The patient has the right to receive from his physician the necessary information to give informed consent before any procedure or treatment is undertaken. The patient also has the right to know the name of the person performing the procedure or treatment.

4. The patient has the right to decline treatment to the extent permitted by law, and to be informed of the medical consequences of his action.

5. The patient has the right to privacy concerning his program of medical care.

6. The patient has the right to expect that all records and communications that pertain to his care shall be kept confidential except as required by law or on the instructions of the patient.

7. The patient has the right to expect that, within its ability, the hospital will make reasonable response to his request for services and must provide evaluation, service, and referral as indicated by the urgency of the case. When medically permissible, a patient may be transferred to another facility only after he, or the appropriate responsible person, if he is unable, has received a complete explanation of the need for, and alternatives to, such a transfer.

8. The patient has the right to receive information about any relationship of this hospital to other health-care and educational institutions, insofar as his care is concerned.

9. The patient has the right to be advised if a hospital staff member or group proposes to engage him in human experimentation, and he has the right to refuse to participate.

10. The patient has the right to expect reasonable continuing care and to be informed by his physician of his health-care needs following his discharge from the hospital.

11. The patient has the right to examine and receive an explanation of his bill, regardless of the source of payment.

12. The patient has the right to know which hospital rules and regulations apply to his conduct as a patient.

The Operation

Prior to surgery, certain medications are withheld—diuretics, for example, because of the fear of loss of potassium. Low potassium levels in the blood can cause the heart to beat erratically. The beta-blockers are continued, as are medications used to regulate the heart rhythm. Some surgeons administer *dipyridamole (Persantine)* before the operation to inhibit platelets from forming clots in the new grafts. (These are continued after surgery along with aspirin, if there are no contraindications.)

The physical therapist's instructions before and after surgery will consist of teaching the patient how to breathe with his diaphragm, how to breathe when the chest is splintered, and how to cough. There is also a psychiatric nurse who comes to visit the patient to determine his mental status. This has several important benefits to the patient after the operation, as there are post-operative changes that occur in some people.

During the night before the operation, the patient is prepped and cleansed with a special soap, especially the chest and abdomen. The legs will be shaved in order to keep a sterile field. Sometimes, no later than 9:00 P.M., a small snack may be given, but from then on, nothing further is taken by mouth, except slight sips of water, to be given with a sedative prior to sleep.

On the morning of the operation, the patient is generally

given a sedative, which might be intramuscular morphine. The operation is generally performed in the morning, although if there is heavy scheduling, it may occur later in the day. The patient will be taken to the operating room on a stretcher, feeling quite drowsy, where the surgical team will be waiting. The team normally includes the anesthesiologist, the surgeon, the surgical assistants, the nurses, and the cardiopulmonary technicians.

The operating room for open-heart surgery is larger than most because it has to accommodate a lot of equipment and a staff of at least nine or ten. Besides the operating table, equipment includes overhead lights, instrument tables, and tables that hold the gauze, the pads, the sponges, and the dressing and bandages during the operation. The heart-lung machine will be close to the operating table, attended by the technicians, and will take over the work of the heart (pumping blood to the organs) so the heart can be operated on. An array of electronic devices includes television sets that display the electrocardiogram, arterial blood pressure, and temperature.

The surgeon, as the leader of the team, is in command at all times. Prior to entering the operating room, he may again review the X-ray films of the patient's coronary arteries. It is he who issues the direction to the pump team to go on bypass, and once its work is completed, he prepares to take the patient off bypass. Bypass means that the heart function is taken over by the machine.

There are generally two senior residents and surgical assistants. The surgical assistants work with the surgeon during the operation and are a useful second and third pair of hands (and on occasion even more assistance will be available to the surgeon). The nurse is called a scrub nurse because, like the surgeon, she has direct contact with the patient and the instruments. The scrub nurse sets up the instruments and all the equipment on the table before the start of the operation. There is also a circulating nurse, also known as the operating room manager, who sees that everything is in its proper place. Heart-lung experts operate the machine that is essential for the support of the life of the patient during at least one-third of the operation.

An intravenous line is placed and the anesthesiologist inserts medication. The breathing tube (the endotracheal tube) is placed through the sleeping patient's mouth and into his windpipe. This is attached to a breathing machine, which regulates the breathing of the patient. When the anesthesia is administered, a catheter is placed into the bladder to measure and drain the urine. This helps the surgeon to evaluate the function of the kidneys (the catheter generally remains in place for a day or two after surgery). Another line is placed in an artery in the wrist or groin, and two lines into the large veins of the shoulder area. These are further connections to monitors that record the blood pressure in the arteries and veins. The oxygen content of the blood is ascertained periodically from the line that is in the artery. The pressure in the large veins is measured by the intravenous line. The work of the heart is measured by another tube that is placed in the pulmonary artery. All the information that is displayed on the television screens is under the constant scrutiny of the physicians and nurses.

The heart-lung machine will take over the breathing and the blood circulation during the entire surgery. This machine takes the blood from the patient's veins and returns it to the heart, where it receives oxygen; removes the carbon dioxide; and returns it back to the arterial side. It is a spinning roller pump that pushes five to six quarts of blood every minute. Heparin, which you will recall is an anti-coagulant, is infused into the blood just before the patient is connected to the heart-lung machine, to prevent the blood from clotting.

After the chest is properly painted with antiseptic, the

surgeon makes an incision fourteen to sixteen inches long, depending on how large the patient is, down the center of the chest. The skin is separated, bringing into view the sternum, and the ribs are gently wedged apart, held open by metal retractors. The first thing that the surgeon sees is the thin sac that protects the heart, called the pericardium, which is pinkish in color. If there is a lot of fat, the color will be yellow. An ice-cold saline solution is poured over the the heart to cool it. The heart is gently lifted so a cardiac "jock-strap" can be wrapped around it to give it support that will keep it still while the surgeon operates.

If the saphenous vein is used, it is removed after an incision on the inside of the leg that runs from the lower half to somewhere above the knee. The length is determined by the number of bypasses needed. Each bypass needs approximately seven inches of vein. The surgeon removes a longer segment than he will probably need so that there will be more to work with. If still more is needed, the incision in the leg will be extended.

The scrub nurse will hand the vein to the surgeon. The vein will be inspected by the surgeon to be certain there are no varicosities, because if there are, the surgeon may choose not to use it. (This vein can be removed without any risk. Usually, there is no residual loss for the patient.)

After the vein is removed, a small rubber tube is left in place in the leg to drain any fluid that may accumulate in the wound, and the leg is bandaged. The aorta is then isolated with a special clamp, and a small hole is made in it so that one end of the saphenous vein can be sewn in. An incision is made in the diseased coronary artery below the blockage, and the other end of the vein graft is then attached to the opening. This is repeated for each vessel.

In the case of the internal mammary arteries, a similar procedure is used. When this is completed, the patient's body becomes rewarmed by raising the temperature of the water in the heart-lung machine. Some wires are attached directly to the heart and attached to a pacemaker in case the heart rate suddenly drops. It is a safeguard so that when the patient comes off bypass surgery his heart, if necessary, can be activated mechanically. Following the operation, which may last four to five hours, the chest is sutured and the patient is brought to the special intensive care unit. There, monitoring continues, and often the patient receives intravenous nitroglycerine to prevent the other arteries and the new grafts from going into spasm. Blood pressure, breathing, temperature, and color are continuously monitored, and in anywhere from twelve to twenty-four hours the patient leaves the operating room. He is alert at this time and is encouraged to breathe deeply and to cough up all the secretions from his lungs. In many cardiac centers, patients are given Persantine three or four times a day in order to prevent clots from forming in the new channels.

Once the breathing tube is removed, you begin to drink fluids and progressively are advanced to a full meal. In a few days, you will be able to care for some of your own personal needs. The stay in the hospital is approximately a week or two. It takes a month or so for the breastbone to heal completely, and you can anticipate returning to work within six to eight weeks. The incision changes from purple to read, and eventually to the normal color, and in a year, many people can barely see their incision.

As a rule, a physical therapist will be included in the post-operative care, with exercises beginning as soon as you return to your room. At first, exercise may consist of sitting in a chair; this will be followed by walking around the room and down the hall. Each person has an individual rehabilitation plan and will progress at a different rate.

After bypass surgery, many surgeons will place the patient on two aspirins a day and prescribe Persantine four times a day. Some of the medications that were given before the surgery might be restarted, depending upon the individual case.

Complications from the operation are uncommon. They are mostly nuisances. Infections do occur, and if they are promptly recognized and treated, will not slow or halt the recovery. The most disagreeable part of the operation is from the pains of the operation, in the chest where it was split, and the constant nagging feeling of a pulling sensation in the leg where the veins were removed. The more the patient cooperates with the nursing staff and the physical therapist on coughing and keeping the lungs clear and breathing deeply, the less likely are complications like pneumonia to occur.

Complications of Coronary Bypass Surgery

Any operation, no matter how minor, can have complications. Going to a dentist and having peridontal work done can cause infections and abscesses. Having a tooth pulled can cause hemorrhage and infection. It has to be accepted that serious complications of bypass surgery also exist, but they are uncommon. Some estimates have indicated that approximately 50 percent of those undergoing bypass surgery suffer some degree of complications, even though there are certain fewer serious complications as we develop knowledge and technique.

Dr. George Crile, chairman of the Cleveland Hospital department of surgery, is quoted as saying, "Small hospitals which do only a few bypass operations a year may have more mortality rate, as compared to medical centers where surgeons have a great deal of experience."

But regardless how skilled the surgeon and how superb the facilities, complications such as a heart attack do occur. Heart attacks can occur before surgery, when the patient is connected to the heart lung machine, or after surgery.

Those patients who have left main artery disease, poor left ventricular function, and arteriosclerosis in their distal vessels have more of a propensity to develop a heart attack.

In a recent case study on arterial surgery, a heart attack occurred in 23 of the 357 patients, or 6.4 percent. The percentage may vary. Dr. Nicholas Kouchoukoss, at the University of Alabama, reported that 5 percent of their patients suffered a heart attack during bypass surgery. The news is not all bad, because most of these heart attacks were not fatal. If a heart attack has occurred, it might require a little longer stay in the intensive care unit.

Dr. René Favalaro, the pioneer in coronary bypass surgery, has stated that the risk of heart attacks depends upon how good the heart is before surgery, the extent of atherosclerosis, and the operative technique. On rare occasion, the patient on the heart-lung machine cannot be taken off, because the heart does not re-start. The number of hearts that cannot be removed from the machine has been approximated in the vicinity of 3,000 a year, and it is these patients who might someday be candidates for an artificial heart, followed by heart transplant.

LUNG COMPLICATIONS AFTER SURGERY

Cigarette smokers, who generate much mucus and have damaged lung tissue, are prime candidates to develop pneumonia. After surgery, patients are encouraged to cough and are turned from side to side. Collected mucus can plug the tubes, and bacteria may grow, causing pneumonia.

The normal lung has its own vacuum cleaner (cells called *cilia* are in constant motion, sweeping away secretions), but in a person who has just recovered from anesthesia, the reflexes of coughing and secretion removal are impaired, especially if the chest has been split open. With the excellent lung therapy now administered in recovery rooms, lung complications are diminished.

Phlebitis of the legs is also becoming less common, as patients are swiftly ambulated. Movement of the toes, and bending and straightening the ankles, helps the circulation.

NEUROLOGICAL COMPLICATIONS

A stroke may be precipitated by bypass surgery, especially if there is unknown hardening of the arteries to the brain. Some of the less serious problems consist of minor injuries to the nerves of the arms and legs, which result in temporary tingling; occasionally, a more pronounced effect results, such as hoarseness of the voice, weakness, and drooping of an eyelid. The vast majority recuperate without any permanent damage.

In one study, strokes occurred in 5.2 percent of 421 patients, but were severe in only 2 percent of operated patients. The cause of these strokes is believed to be either a clot traveling to the brain, pre-existing arterial disease of the brain, or an air embolus that travels to and lodges in the brain.

Case: A seventy-two-year-old male underwent a successful bypass operation. The operation was performed because of severe, constant chest pain that could not be relieved any other way. Two days after the operation, he said he "felt fine but I'll need new glasses. My vision is blurred and I see double."

Neurological examination was normal, except that he lost part of his vision, the result of a clot in his occipital lobe, the back of his brain. No other neurological loss occurred, and the patient's vision did improve.

PSYCHOLOGICAL FACTORS

Surgery some times produces some psychiatric changes; it is surprising that they do not occur more often. Being placed in a totally foreign environment with tubes in your arms, urinary tract, and throat is understandably frightening to many. There is a break in the circadian rhythm of the body. Normal sleep is disturbed since the lights are continuously bright; night and day become merged into one in the surgical intensive care unit. With the coughing exercises, the constant monitoring, and the periodic examinations, it is difficult for persons to sleep. The medications themselves can cause fatigue, disorientation, and even hallucinations.

Case: James decided to have coronary bypass surgery. Although he was cautioned to stop smoking prior to the operation, he actually increased the consumption of his cigarettes. He also wanted to be certain that everything was in order prior to undergoing surgery, so he rushed around, handling last-minute details on his job and his home, speaking to his lawyer, setting his will straight, talking to people who had the operation, checking on his surgeon.

Prior to James's operation, he was given physical therapy and was interviewed by a psychiatric nurse to ascertain his attitudes and fears. The nurse wrote in the chart: "Understands the operation and feels optimistic, and he doesn't have any undue fears, but is very anxious."

He quickly developed some complications, with his lung deteriorated, as he accumulated a great deal of mucus and developed pneumonia. An electrocardiogram taken after the operation disclosed that he had had a heart attack during the operation. His stay was prolonged in the intensive care unit because he developed another complication, which is rather common, an irregular heartbeat. The irregular heartbeat was swiftly treated with digitalis.

When he was finally moved out of the intensive care unit, his wife noted that he had become much more quiet than usual. He said very little. Whereas before the operation he was somewhat fearful and anxious, now he was calm, as if sedated. The doctor checked the chart and found he was not receiving any medications for sedation.

He went home at the end of the twelfth day, feeling worn out, as if "a truck ran over me." His recovery was not as rapid as expected. He refused to enter a rehabilitation program because he felt too weak and tired. All the signs pointed to the fact that James was suffering from post-operative depression, a rather common complication of operations, especially bypass surgery. Once he was convinced that his operation was a success and that he would have a fresh start, his depression lifted.

Comment: Sometimes patients benefit from counseling if the depression persists. Depression has numerous causes, including chemical imbalances in the brain, medications, situational factors, and major trauma. Psychiatrists call this last a post-traumatic depression, recognized in some war veterans, car and plane crash victims, and those suffering other near-death events.

CHEST PAIN

There are three major types of chest pain that can occur in the first two weeks after bypass:

One pain is consistently present, arising from the incision. It is a nagging, pulling, sticking, pinching feeling, which will eventually disappear.

A second kind, present in perhaps one of ten people, is due to the heart covering's becoming inflamed, a condition called *pericarditis.* This pain characteristically is worsened by breathing. The doctor swiftly recognizes the origin of this pain with the stethoscope from the sounds, described as two pieces of leather being rubbed together (pericardial friction rub). This annoying pain resolves with anti-inflammatory medications.

A third kind of pain results from the graft closing—the reappearance of angina—which may have the same characteristics as the chest pain before surgery.

A thallium stress test is performed to pinpoint the origin of the chest pain, or coronary angiography may be used before discharge. Anti-anginal medications are reinstituted, and if no relief is obtained, angioplasty or surgery is considered.

Less common causes of chest pain after bypass surgery include pneumonia and pulmonary embolus, and inflammation of the esophagus and stomach.

THE DARK SIDE OF CORONARY ARTERY SURGERY

Besides the complications of surgery that I have listed, there is a small number of patients who become worsened by the operation. Not only can grafts close, but the heart function can deteriorate further.

Some patients suffer from chronic congestive heart failure as a result of the surgery. The heart muscle, becoming damaged during the operation, loses its ability to contract. Persons living under these conditions require an abundance of medication to rid them of accumulated fluid in the lungs. Their hearts are too damaged to be repaired, and these patients may be candidates for heart transplantation.

9

Life after Bypass Surgery

WITH your new blood vessels, the quality of life should be better than before the operation. The dreadful pain of angina not controlled with the medications will have only a 10 percent chance of surfacing again.

A good part of how well you do will depend on attitude —optimism, confidence, a will to surge forward to a constructive life. Rehabilitation begins in the hospital, taught by the cardiac rehabilitation team, and continues at home.

There are some general rules to follow after surgery in order to reduce the strain on the heart. Avoid bending at the waist, since this increases the pressure in the abdomen and transmits it to the heart. Weight-lifting, pushing, pulling, and straining are discouraged in the early weeks after surgery. I prefer that patients not drive a car for at least four weeks, because it takes that long for the breastbone to heal, and a sudden jarring of the chest against the steering wheel can interfere with its healing process. Each rehabilitation program is individually tailored by the doctor, and below are general principles that patients must check with their doctor.

A progressive, useful program is to walk five minutes, a quarter of a mile, once a day for several days, and then five minutes twice daily for two or three days. If there is no fatigue, you can gradually increase your walking time at a leisurely pace, to ten minutes, one-half mile, once daily, and then ten minutes twice daily for four to five days. Then walk fifteen minutes, three-quarters of a mile, once daily, and continue doing that for several days. Finally, increase the time and the pace to thirty minutes, two miles, once daily. The patient should judge each progression of activity by how he feels. If there is chest pain or shortness of breath, dizziness, or much fatigue, he should discontinue the program and inform his physician. The walking should not be done in the very cold or very hot weather, and should not be done if he is tired or upset, or after eating. If showering after exercise, the water should be lukewarm and not cold or very hot. Sudden hot or cold water can cause the heart to beat irregularly. Before leaving the hospital, more specific instructions will be given by the surgeon and with the physical therapist.

The most important goal in the treatment and the rehabilitation program is to eliminate fear—the fear of harming oneself and the fear of dying. A positive state of mind is probably the best healer. After four weeks or so, the patient may return to part-time work. After all, the purpose of the operation in the first place was to bring the patient back to a normal life.

Patients are urged to follow a low-cholesterol diet and not to smoke, in order to prevent further clogging of arteries and the progression of their arteriosclerosis. Cholesterol intake should come down to a level of 200 mg per day. Two to four ounces of alcohol is permitted, and as a matter of fact, is encouraged. A pleasing quiet dinner with candlelight and wine has a much more salutary effect than a tranquilizer.

Sexual activity is encouraged and can be resumed as soon as you are capable of climbing two flights of stairs. A true and humorous story comes to mind:

One of my more sexually ambitious patients asked about when he might return to lovemaking. I explained to him that his pulse rate during sexual activity rises to approximately 110, which is the equivalent to climbing two flights of stairs, and that he could now resume his sexual activity, since it was several weeks since he had returned home.

"I know," he said, "but my wife doesn't believe me. Would you please write on your prescription pad that I may resume sexual activity?"

He returned the following week, distressed and much dismayed, and said, "My wife still doesn't believe me. Could you do me a favor and write another prescription and address it, "To whom it may concern'?"

Some patients suffer unpleasant psychological results from the surgery. One is the fear of doing any activity, as the person thinks it might break the graft open, split the chest, or precipitate another heart attack. It takes a great deal of convincing that this is not going to happen.

Depression, as we saw in James's case, is another not uncommon aftermath of any operation. Some patients who develop a post-traumatic depression experience fear, difficulty in concentration, some memory loss, and nightmares.

Anger and frustration are two non-productive and detrimental emotions. They stimulate the brain to form chemicals (*catecholamines* and *vasopressor*, for example) that elevate the blood pressure, raise the pulse, and play havoc with the vascular system. Tension makes some people feel bloated and swollen because they retain water. Heart failure, strokes, hypertension crises—all are at times triggered by emotional stress. After bypass surgery, these destructive emotions delay recovery and are in part responsible for chest pains which surface.

Case: A forty-seven-year-old male who had had a heart attack continued to have chest pain. Prior to his heart attack, there was enormous tension at work. He felt life should have treated him more squarely, that he should have advanced to become manager. Everyone around him was an idiot, misjudged him—they were all doing everything wrong. "Nobody wants to work except me," he said, "and I have to carry the burden of five lazy people."

It was with this attitude that he arrived at the coronary care unit. It was discovered that he had a left main artery stenosis of greater than 85 percent and continual chest pain, and he had bypass. The surgery was successful, but in the surgical intensive care unit and later, everything hurt him, the odors were unbearable, the sounds were irritating, and he needed a great deal of narcotics to ease the pain in his chest from the incision. His cantankerous attitude continued; he was discharged from the hospital but fiercely resisted returning to work because of intolerable pain in his chest and his thighs. Also, painkillers were making him groggy. Finally, after many months of reassurance and cajoling, he returned to work.

One month later, he was again back in the hospital with chest pain, which he claimed was the same pain as before the operation. He had another cardiac catheterization, which revealed all the grafts were open, and he again returned to work, and four weeks later, was re-admitted into the hospital because of chest pain. "They just don't understand the pressure on me. My boss requires me to do work that I just can't do."

Now, several years later, he is still working but is considering taking a disability pension. His hands are still moist, he trembles and stutters, loses his temper easily, has reverted back to smoking, and has regained weight. He is in the same position, if not worse, than before his bypass surgery.

Comment: Without the proper attitude and desire, without the willingness to change destructive behavior, the rehabilitative benefits of bypass surgery may be very short-lived.

A resetting of your psychic thermostat is an important part of a good and prolonged recovery. Values are re-examined, and there should be a search for a more meaningful life. A sharpening up of your senses for appreciation of the beauty of the world, rather than focusing on the underside of life, is regarded by many as essential. Most patients develop a wholesome new philosophical outlook on their own lives and goals and are gratified to be alive and working.

After bypass surgery, angina will return in 5 percent of patients a year; in approximately two-thirds of those with recurrent angina this is due to closure of the vein graft, and in the other one-third to progression of disease in the remaining arteries. Most physicians agree that the clogging of the graft occurs because of persistent elevations of blood lipids and poor control of such other risk factors as obesity, hypertension, and smoking.

The return-to-work-incentive does not work well following many bypass operations. In one study of eight hundred patients surveyed after heart surgery, two-thirds had anxiety, depression, confusion, and feelings of unreality. Seventeen percent claimed that psychological factors interfered with their recovery and return to work. Some patients become socially limited and rely on their families and friends to do everything for them. If one of the reasons for having bypass surgery is to return the patient to work—and it is—it seems to fail in some 40 percent of the cases. In some other studies psychological impairments occurred in 16 percent.

There is conflicting data on the number of people who actually return to work after bypass surgery. In one study, W.D. Johnson and his colleagues followed 2,229 male patients for as long as ten years. The main reasons for not working were physical disability, confirmed by the physician. Older patients had a tendency to retire early. Thirty percent of all the older patients said that the desire to relax was the main reason for not working.

In another study by J.E. Dimsdale and colleagues, it was discovered that 40 percent were returning to the same job, and 19 percent had more demanding jobs. The various studies showed a return to work varying from 20 to 60 percent. All the studies proved a disappointing return-to-work rate after surgery. The reasons cited varied from fatigue, chest pain, and "I had enough" to lack of financial motivation (i.e., they did not need to work). The average percentage of patients returned to work: about 60 percent in the first year, 56 percent at four years, and 53 percent at five years. Patients who sustain heart attacks and have no bypass surgery have a significant higher percentage of return to work.

Questions Asked

"*Will I no longer have to take any medications?*" If there is no reappearance of angina, there will be no need to take the medications taken prior to surgery. There is a 20 percent chance that the chest pain may occur again. Most cardiologists feel two aspirins a day plus Persantine should be given to help to prevent the reclogging of the veins. Medications that were used for an irregular heartbeat such as atrial fibrillation are continued.

"*Will I have to stay on a low-cholesterol diet?*" The answer is Yes, in my opinion.

"*Is my heart now normal?*" The answer is that the heart muscle may or may not have been normal before the operation, and if it was, the likelihood is that it will remain so. The purpose of the operation was to preserve the integrity of the muscle. If the heart muscle was abnormal before the operation, there is a chance that its function will improve because it now has a new supply of blood, but it is likely it will still be abnormal.

"*Can I still get a heart attack?*" The answer is Yes.

"*Will I miss the veins taken from the leg?*" Removing the veins will not affect the state of your legs except for some periodic minor aching or swelling.

"*Will I be able to play tennis/jog/play squash/swim, and so on again as I did before the operation?*" If the patient is completely rehabilitated and has entered into a good exercise program, there is no reason not to be able to play tennis. Patients are encouraged to return to the type of physical activity they enjoy most.

"*Do I have to stay on a low-salt diet like the one I was given in the hospital?*" A low-salt diet is preferable in most instances, especially if there is a propensity for high blood pressure. A low-salt diet is mandatory if there has been complete heart failure.

"*If my new channels get blocked again, will I have to be re-operated on?*" Most surgeons will agree that between the seventh and tenth year, 60 percent of the channels may get blocked again, and re-operation will be necessary if symptoms reappear. Re-operation has more of a risk than the first operation, but it is being performed throughout the country. Angioplasty might very well come to substitute for re-operation. At the present time, some patients with graft closure are being reopened with the balloon dilation. Graft closure was more common in the earlier years of surgery when the technique was not as refined as today and our knowledge of prevention was not as full. Closure of the graft may be delayed even more now that we are using aspirin and Persantine and substituting the internal mammary artery for the leg veins when possible.

"*Will irregular heartbeats be corrected by by pass surgery?*" Doctors now realize that palpitations, or extra beats, generally do not cause any problems in a person with a normal heart. "I feel like my heart is doing somersaults" or "My heart is going to jump out of my chest" are some of the ways patients describe palpitations. Still others say, "I feel my heart beat" or "It beats so hard I want to faint."

These palpitations are usually caused by anxiety: anxiety causes adrenaline to flow and stimulates the heart to skip a beat. Medical students before an examination have been found to have frequent extra heartbeats, which are called *premature ventricular contractions* (PVCs). Driving in New York City traffic, coffee, cigarettes, watching a football game, all are stimuli that can result in palpitations.

Coronary artery disease can cause extra beats if the circulation to the heart is perturbed and the natural pacemaker of the heart is irritated. Coronary bypass surgery may or may not correct abnormal heart rhythms. The irregular beating of a heart is not an indication to perform bypass surgery.

Case: A forty-eight-year-old man had skipped beats of his heart most of his life. He recalls playing basketball as a youngster and feeling his heart thumping. He went to see his physician when he was forty-six, still complaining of the extra beats. The physical examination disclosed a 175-pound, 5′8″ man whose blood pressure was 140/80 and pulse 70. The heart examination was normal. An electrocardiogram did, however, disclose some extra abnormal heartbeats. The patient underwent a stress test and many extra beats appeared, and there was one episode of four ventricular beats almost simultaneously *(ventricular tachycardia).* The test was stopped and the patient was advised to have cardiac catheterization and angiography, which disclosed that he had a left anterior descending artery narrowed by 75 percent. The doctor feared that he might have a heart attack and advised the patient to have bypass surgery.

The left anterior descending artery was bypassed, but

after the operation the patient experienced serious extra heartbeats. Medication was given, which included Pronestyl and Inderal, and the extra beats disappeared. The patient was discharged from the hospital with the medications, and as the months went on, he felt very well; however, his extra beats reappeared whenever he had tension. He eliminated coffee and cigarettes and increased his physical activity. He learned relaxation techniques, which decreased his palpitations, and he eventually was able to stop all medications.

Comment: This patient demonstrates that extra beats are not always resolved by bypass surgery.

IV

TECHNOLOGICAL FRONTIERS

10

Pacemakers

ALL human beings have their own internal pacemaker, which enables the heart to contract normally, pumping ten pints of blood every minute. This specialized electrical system generates the impulses for cardiac contraction within special cells, called pacemaker cells, which are grouped at the uppermost part of the pacemaker cells, which are grouped at the uppermost part of the heart (the *SA node*), sends signals through special tracts to another point (the *AV node*), and divides into branches supplying the right and left ventricles. The signals flow smoothly, but occasionally they are interrupted or stimulated by a variety of agents, such as coffee, alcohol, and pipe and cigarette smoking, or by too little oxygen in an otherwise healthy individual, as, for example, in carbon monoxide poisoning. The interruption or the extra impulses cause the sensation of a skipped beat or an extra beat, or a feeling of "my heart is turning in my chest," referred to as palpitation. The transmission of this electricity through the branches normally makes the heart contract between 60 and 85 beats per minute. The pulse rate, synonymous with the heart beat, may vary from individual to individual. Some people may have normal pulse beats of 45 and 50 all their lives. Athletes tend to have lower pulse rates. Children have a faster pulse rate than young adults, and the aged have slower pulse beats.

What Is a Pacemaker?

In 1872, the first heart was paced by Dr. Guillaume-Benjamin Armand Duchene. He used rhythmic electrical stimulation of the chest in order to resuscitate patients who had collapsed. This technique consisted of two electrodes, one placed in a stationary position on the patient's body, the other, stimulating electrode, held by Dr. Duchene, moved to different parts of the heart. Duchene actually resuscitated a twenty-year-old female whose heart went into complete chaotic irregular heartbeat (ventricular fibrillation). The woman was successfully resuscitated more than one hundred years ago.

The earliest pacemakers consisted of electrodes with a power source attached to the skin. This was highly unsatisfactory, causing severe burns. In November of 1956, the first electrode was placed into the heart muscle by Dr. Henry Bahnson of Johns Hopkins University. Dr. Walter Lilleihei, also of Johns Hopkins, and his team then continued to work on the placement of artificial pacemakers.

In the United States, approximately 200,000 people live with implanted pacemakers. It has been estimated that in the next ten years, another 100,000 will have their hearts paced by an artificial internal device. The average pacemaker recipient is seventy-two years of age and has an additional life expectancy of twelve years. Women who wear pacemakers have an average life expectancy considerably longer. Eighty percent of the pacemaker population is over fifty-five. It has been estimated that one out of 300 persons over fifty-five years of age, or one out of every 1,500 of the total population, carries an implanted pacemaker.

The pacemaker is a small electrical unit, about the size of

a cigarette package (we apologize for that dirty word), containing batteries that produce impulses to make the heart beat. A long electrode connects the battery to the right side of the heart. The pacemaker is preset for a particular pulse rate.

The earliest pacemakers were inserted by actually opening the chest wall and implanting them in the heart. By 1965, pacemakers were inserted by threading a wire through an arm or shoulder vein, since it was found that going through the chest wall was no longer necessary. Pacemaker wires are placed in the right side of the heart and the pacemaker unit is placed on the surface of the chest. During open-heart surgery, a precautionary standby pacemaker wire is inserted, ready to be used if necessary.

Under fluoroscopic control, an opening is made in the vein and the electrode is passed into the right side of the heart. The electrode is attached to the sensor device, which is placed in a skin pocket constructed in front of the chest. The anatomic and functional position is confirmed with the fluoroscope, and for the next twenty-four to forty-eight hours, the patient is monitored by electrocardiogram to be certain that the electrode does not get displaced, as it does in 5 to 10 percent of patients. A chest X-ray is taken at that time to confirm the position of the pacemaker. These pacemakers are called permanent pacemakers, in contradistinction to temporary pacemakers, which are frequently used in a coronary care unit when a very slow heartbeat occurs, as sometimes is the case after a heart attack.

Indications for Pacemaker Use

When the conduction becomes completely interrupted and the ventricles beat independently from the rest of the heart, we speak of a complete *heart block.* The pulse may then be 35 or less. In some of these instances the heart is not only beating slowly, it may periodically stop and then restart. This sudden slowing of the heart to a pulse rate of below 40, or the sudden arrest of the heart, can cause a patient to collapse, have dizzy spells, fainting spells, and a variety of neurological symptoms, ranging from double vision to headaches and seizures. Chronic fatigue, poor exercise abilities, and, on occasion, sudden death may result. Therefore, when the heart's pacemaker fails—because of a heart attack or sclerosis, infection, injuries, and so forth—an artificial pacemaker must be inserted, a pacemaker that will now take over the job of stimulating the heart.

It must be fully documented that the patient does indeed have a heart block with a resultant slow pulse or episodes of cardiac standstill. Casual listening to the heartbeat and examining the patient will not provide sufficient evidence of the patient's need for a pacemaker. Most centers throughout the United States require a cardiologist to confirm the diagnosis with appropriate testing before referring the patient to the surgeon.

Pacemakers should not be inserted unless proper follow-up care can be provided. Surveillance systems needed to check the workings of the pacemaker range from simple periodic monitoring of an electrocardiographic rhythm strip to comprehensive clinics providing detailed study. It is possible to test the competency of the pacemaker over the telephone. Central pacemaker stations are located all over the United States. Pacemaker recipients can transmit their heartbeats over the telephone by attaching a few wires to their body and placing the other end to a telephone receiver. Each system may vary from pacemaker to pacemaker. If pacemaker surveillance cannot be provided, the patient should either get another surgeon or refuse to have a pacemaker. It needs to be re-emphasized that the biggest problem of pacemaker insertion is trying to document that the dizziness, fainting, or weak spells are caused by the heart and not something else.

The patient must also recognize that the unit itself, or the battery, will be placed underneath the skin, and that there will be a bulge evident. Females, rightfully, will be concerned about their appearance in a bathing suit or with a low decolletage. Surgeons will try to take into consideration the cosmetic needs of the individual patient.

When the physician advises the insertion of a pacemaker, the patient should respond: "How do you know?" I strongly urge a second opinion if the patient's heart has not been monitored for at least a twenty-four-hour period. The monitoring system can be accomplished by a device called the Holter monitor, which the patient carries a sling over his shoulder, the electrodes attached to the surface of his body. The patient keeps an accurate record of the times when he feels dizzy or weak or has other symptoms, which is later corroborated by the tape of the recording of the patient's heart. If it indeed demonstrates episodes of complete standstill of the heart or very slow pulse beats while the patient is symptomatic, then the pacemaker should be inserted. Monitoring with a continuous electrocardiogram in a hospital for several days is as good, if not better. A cardiac stress test may also be helpful in revealing any irregularities of the heart.

A very slow pulse rate of 40 or 38 in a completely asymptomatic patient may not necessarily warrant a pacemaker, unless it occurs with a patient who definitely has an abnormal heart, secondary to a heart attack, infection, or rheumatic heart disease. In these situations a pacemaker might be considered prophylactically. Although pacemakers do not prevent heart attacks or inhibit hardening of the arteries, they are critically involved with the electrical conduction of the heart. A pacemaker is not a substitute for bypass surgery.

Recently, a new type of pacemaker is being used, called the dual-chamber pacing. This pacemaker has the advantage of making the heart work more efficiently as it paces the heart in the usual normal sequence: impulses starting from the atrium and then going to the ventricle.

These new pacemakers are $4,000 more expensive and are presently being evaluated to determine if the extra cost is warranted, especially in the elderly patient.

11

Secondhand Hearts

The Heart Transplant

LEWIS Washkansky, a fifty-four-year-old diabetic, was suffering from terminal heart disease at the Groote-Schuur Hospital in Capetown, South Africa. One night, his lungs filled with water and his legs became swollen—his heart was barely able to force blood from its chambers. On the same night, December 2, 1967, a twenty-four-year-old woman who had suffered multiple injuries was dying. In the early hours of the morning of December 3d, in the adjoining operating theater, after the young girl's brain injuries were found to be beyond treatment, she was certified dead and connected to a heart machine that cooled the body to 26° Centrigrade (79° Fahrenheit). The cooled heart with the aortic clamp was removed gently, placed in a bowl of physiological solution, and carried swiftly to the other operating room. All of this took place within four minutes. At the same time, at 3:01 A.M. precisely, the heart of Lewis Washkansky was removed. The young girl's heart was trimmed to be sure it was the right fit and sutured in place, and the body of Washkansky was re-warmed. His second-hand heart was electrically shocked and it began to beat. Someone called the medical superintendent and said, "Sir, we have just transplanted a heart and the patient is well."

Miraculously, the signs of heart failure disappeared: the water-swollen legs returned to their normal state, the liver decreased in size, the lungs were free of water, and it became apparent on this historic day that it was possible to receive a second-hand heart and survive. Although the survival lasted only thirteen days—the patient died from infection, secondary to pneumonia—the heart itself had continued to pump.

On January 2, 1968, Dr. Christiaan Barnard performed a second heart transplantation, this time on Philip Bleiberg, a dentist, who lived for 593 days.

The age of the Frankenstein monster had arrived. Secondhand hearts, livers, lungs, bone marrows—and in the not-too-distant future, brains! From that moment on, heart transplantations were performed all over the world, and by 1969, 143 were reported. The longest survivor was a forty-five-year-old French priest: operated on May 12, 1968; died October 17, 1969.

Skeptics abounded, and moral and ethical questions were raised concerning timing of death and when the heart should be removed from the donor and from the recipient. The major problem of heart transplantations remained the rejection of the donor organs. Antibodies formed against the donor organs and sometimes the organs could not long survive. Recently, however, an effective immunosuppressant drug, called *cyclosporin,* has been discovered, which has given new impetus to the transplant program.

Heart transplantation is not new. It was first performed, on dogs, by Professor Alex Carrel, a French biologist who won the Nobel Prize for physiology and medicine in 1912. It was accomplished with the stump of the donor's heart attached to the dog's artery, through the neck, and the heart did pump for an hour in that fashion.

Even further back, a cultured, but perhaps overly-zealous, Chinese doctor of the third century B.C., by the name of Pien Ch-iao, administered sleeping potions to groups of soldiers, and after they had fallen into a drunken stupor, opened up their chests and stole some of the organs, including their hearts. Unsuccessfully, he tried to transplant these organs. The unwitting donors, clearly, did not survive this audacious experiment.

There are other legends, throughout history, about transplantation—for example, the famous tale of the two brothers, Cosmas and Damian, the patron saints of surgery. The legend holds that one of the brothers removed the cancerous leg of a white man and replaced it with that of a recently killed Moor. The following morning, the white man awoke with one white leg and one brown leg.

The first American heart transplant took place at University Hospital at the Mississippi Medical Center, but it failed. The donor's heart came from a chimpanzee and not from another human being. The operation was performed by Dr. James Hardy, then from the University of Mississippi.

Dr. Norman Shumway, at the Stanford, California, Medical School on January 6, 1968, transplanted the heart of a forty-three-year-old woman into Michael Kasperak, who had terminal heart disease. Two days later, the kidneys and the liver failed, and the patient died. At the same time, the British started their heart transplant program, led by Dr. Donald Ross at the National Heart Hospital in London.

By 1970, Dr. Denton Cooley, at St. Luke's Hospital in Houston, Texas, had added an impressive number of heart transplants—twenty—to his credit. (He had performed his first heart transplant on May 3, 1968.)

Since 1968, 640 heart transplants have been performed in this country, and the longest survival has been for fourteen years. Two hundred and eighty-eight patients have received heart transplants at the Stanford Hospital under the auspices of Dr. Shumway. One hundred and twenty-one are still alive. The current one-year survival rate after heart transplant is 88 percent. Patients today have a 50 percent chance of surviving for five years. (In 1968, only 22 percent survived the first year and heart transplantation was generally in disfavor; indeed, by 1972, Stanford was practically the only center left in the pursuit of transplant goals.)

It has been estimated that there may be as many as 30,000 candidates for heart transplantation. These candidates have irreversible heart disease that cannot be treated with medication, valve replacement, or bypass surgery. The criteria for selecting the recipient are that he should be no older than fifty-five, he has to have no underlying kidney, neurological, or blood disorder, and he must be free of lung disease or cancer. Psychiatrically, the recipient must be a well-adjusted individual who can live in surroundings that will make it possible for most careful follow-up.

Heart donors, after accidents, are registered in a heart transplantation clearinghouse. The recipient's blood type ideally should be the same as the donor's. When a heart becomes available, and a recipient has been selected, the recipient's heart team is notified, and one of the surgeons is dispatched to carry the cooled heart to the center where the transplantation is to be performed. As there are more potential recipients than donors, the selection process is extraordinarily difficult.

Some authorities claim that most patients who are given a choice between receiving a new heart or death choose to die. It is common practice that the physician does not tell the patient who the donor was. Carrying on any kind of dialogue with the donor's family is also strongly discouraged.

There are numerous problems that the physician has to face, especially when the patient is over 55. The donor has to be at least under the age of forty, and has to have died from an accident to the brain and not from a cardiac problem. The timing of the transplantation is critical. The human heart cannot, as of this time, survive more than four hours outside the body.

A heart transplantation costs approximately $100,000. Insurance companies are presently deciding whether this procedure will be covered. The federal government, through Medicaid, does cover the procedure.

In the next few years heart transplantation will be as common as placing artificial valves, once it is realized that it is not a science fiction experiment but an important form of treatment of irreversible heart disease.

The Artificial Heart

On December 2, 1982, in Salt Lake City, Utah, an artificial heart was placed in the chest of Dr. Barney Clark, a 61-year-old dentist. The significance of this announcement was as world-shaking as when Neil Armstrong walked on the moon.

The idea of having a machine substitute for a heart was entertained in 1812 by Dr. Julien-Jean Cesar la Gallois, who said: "If one could substitute for the heart a kind of injection [of arterial blood], one would succeed easily in maintaining alive indefinitely any part of the body."

Different pumps were designed in the early 1800s. Later came the pump oxygenator, engineered in 1882 by a Dr. Von Schroder. In England, in 1928, Drs. H.H. Dale and E.H. Shuster devised a pump to replace the function of both the right and the left sides of the heart, and it was tried on animals.

In the early 1930s, Charles Lindbergh's sister-in-law was suffering from serious disease of the valve and Dr. Michael DeBakey was thinking of ways of providing support to her heart while she underwent surgery. As early as 1934, he designed a roller pump, which is presently used in all the heart-lung machines. In 1935, he and Dr. Alex Carrel, a French surgeon (who revolutionized surgery of the vascular system by joining vessels end to end), developed a pump oxygenator. They wrote: "We can perhaps dream of removing diseased organs from the body, placing them in the Lindbergh pump, then replacing them in the patient. There [in the pump], the organs could be treated far more energetically than within the organism and, if cured, can be replanted in the patient."

The "robot heart," as it was called by journalists, hit the headlines in 1935, but failed. Then in 1957, in the Cleveland Clinic, Drs. Tetsuzo Akutsu and Wilem Kolff implanted a totally artificial heart in a dog's chest. The dog survived for ninety minutes. Dr. Denton Cooley, in 1969, operated on a forty-seven-year-old man with terminal heart disease, removed his heart and implanted an air pump designed by Dr. Domingo Liotto. This kept the patient alive for sixty-four hours, until he received a donor's heart.

The first artificial implant in a human being, on December 2, 1982, was built on the contributions of all these scientists over the past hundred years.

At Utah, Drs. Robert Jarvik, Don Olsen, Wilhem Kolff, and William DeVries implanted a motor-driven heart in a calf, which survived for thirty-five days. Another implanted calf lived 268 days. The implant failed because the calf outgrew the size of the pump.

The Jarvik–7 heart consists of a polyurethane device with a diaphragm, with four-layer sheets of polyurethane that are infinitely pliable. It is basically an air-driven pump with two separate ventricles with air chambers. Air is pushed in and out of the air chambers, moving the diaphragm. This pneumatic heart-driver is connected to a source of compressed air vacuum and electricity. It is a large bulky instrument that required the first patient, Dr. Clark, to be in close proximity to it, thus severely restricting his mobility. This brave man survived for ninety-two days and then contracted an influenza illness, with vomiting and severe infections, and finally died 112 days after the heart was implanted. He died not as the result of pump failure but of a generalized infection.

The cost of implanting a heart is in the vicinity of $60,000, which is comparable to a heart transplant. There are all sorts of variations that are under study, such as the native heart remaining in place with mechanical pumps inside it, so-called assisted pumping.

When the heart is irreversibly damaged, no angioplasty, bypass surgery, valve surgery, or medications can possibly maintain life; only a new heart can do this.

Who should be the candidates for an artificial heart? Patients over the age of fifty-five should not be candidates. The first group recommended by the Food and Drug Administration consists of those patients who are unable to be weaned from the cardiopulmonary bypass pump following cardiac operations. Approximately two thousand patients—a very small percentage of the total—never leave the operating room. An artificial heart could be implanted in these patients after all other measures fail, while they wait for a heart transplant.

The next group of patients are the 8- to 10,000 who have terminal disease of the heart muscle (*cardiomyopathy*—caused by virus, alcohol, and metabolic and congenital disorders), who can only survive with a new heart.

About one-third of patients who are selected to receive a cardiac transplant die while they wait for someone to donate a heart. The artificial heart can be a temporary form of life support while waiting for a heart transplant. Those patients who are considered to have terminal disease of the heart have been defined according to certain criteria by the American Heart Association:

1. They should not have any correctable surgical lesions, such as valves or coronary arteries that could be replaced.

2. Patients may be male or female, but must be at least eighteen years old.

3. They must show irreversible heart deterioration that does not respond to treatment after eight weeks.

4. The patient, for follow-up care, must live close to a medical center.

5. He or she must have a stable home situation with a reliable spouse, sibling, or other person.

6. There has to be no other serious medical illness, such as kidney failure, stroke, liver disease, blood disease, or lung disease.

The heart is removed, and the artificial heart tubes are put into place. Many surgeons are skeptical regarding this procedure; there are others who applaud it. Dr. DeVries and his associates, who were responsible for the artificial heart implantation on Dr. Clark, are developing a device that will be portable, enabling a patient to be more mobile.

The major problems of the artificial heart transplant concern the other organs' failing, and the onset of infections, hemorrhages, and strokes.

There are moral issues involved about the selection of candidates, since there are more candidates than hearts. There are also ethical issues involved in prolonging life that has ended by virtue of death of the heart, and perhaps prolonging undue suffering at an unreasonable psychological and financial cost. Dr. Clark was made totally aware of all the implications of the experiment. He signed a thirty-page consent form, and signed again the next day, in case he had changed his mind.

Disease of the heart muscle, or cardiomyopathy, is here to stay. As long as we have not found an adequate medical solution, I strongly favor a surgical attempt to prolong the life of a viable individual The selection should be properly based not only on general medical condition, but also on the psychiatric properties of that individual. I see it as a temporary form of treatment, even as bypass surgery is, until preventive measures have once and for all cured heart disease. Prevention will be the final form of treatment in the future, but for the time being, I applaud the work of Dr. DeVries and Dr. Jarvik in their magnificent attempt to help mankind in a fashion not so long ago thought to be the stuff of science fiction.

Medicine is forever moving forward, reaching out, searching, probing to prolong life and to achieve a better quality of life. I remember when the first artificial valve was placed in 1961, and the outcries of many members of the medical community that it would never last and would never work. It took brave and heroic acts of doctors like Dwight Harkin (who went ahead and demonstrated to the world that an artificial valve prolongs life). To forge ahead in a similar fashion, it took brave and heroic acts—by both scientists and patients—to get to where we are today in dealing with coronary artery disease.

To look through a medical journal of even ten years ago is not only to be reminded of how far we've come in medicine, but to be startled by the degree of progressive acceleration. To look back a single year is to become convinced that in that year more was probably discovered, attempted, accomplished than in the previous two years. The pace is as exhilerating as it is challenging, and I wouldn't miss it for the world.

APPENDIX

*Cardiopulmonary Resuscitation (CPR)**

SUDDEN cardiac arrest can be the first sign of coronary artery disease. Patients who have had a heart attack are more vulnerable in the first two months following this disaster. With the use of beta-blockers, channel calcium blockers, and aspirin, along with identification of patients who are prone to cardiac arrest, we should further decrease the incidence of sudden death by 30 to 40 percent.

The mechanism of sudden cardiac arrest is due to an electrical power failure of the heart: the heart goes into ventricular fibrillation. As one pathologist in the early nineteenth century described it, the heart feels like "a bag of twirling worms."

Members of families of heart attack victims, especially a spouse, would do well to learn CPR. Relevant literature reveals that if CPR is initiated by a bystander who witnessed the arrest, the survival rate increased to 43 percent.

Can cardiac arrest by avoided by bypass surgery? The patient with his new channels supplying blood to the heart is less vulnerable to cardiac arrest. Unfortunately, even after patients have bypass surgery, some of them can still go into cardiac arrest, not only because their grafts have closed, but because of electrical short-circuiting of the heart.

Throughout history, many methods of CPR have been devised. In the oldest method, the victim was whipped with stinging nettles, or struck on the skin with hands or wet clothes. Warm ashes, hot water, scalding animal excretions applied to the abdomen or chest—all were thought to be valuable in reviving somebody.

In 1530, Paracelsus, a Swiss chemist and physician, used a fireside bellow to introduce air into the lungs of people who had stopped breathing. This method was used for almost three hundred years. The North American Indians practiced reviving people by blowing smoke into an animal bladder and then into the victim's rectum. Another favorite method was to suspend the victim by his feet with a rope from a tree. This was called the inversion method. Drowning victims were sometimes resuscitated successfully in this manner. Along the waterfront in the United States, the barrel method was used for drowning and intoxicated victims. The victim was placed across an empty bear barrel, the feet were held securely, and the barrel rolled to and fro. Barrel movements forward released pressure on the victim's chest, allowing inspiration, and moving the barrel back caused the body's weight to compress the chest. The Russians had their own method—dashing ice water into the victim's face. The trotting-horse method was used for drowning victims. An unconscious body was placed across the back of a horse and the horse's vigorously moving body compressed the victim's chest and forced out the air; if the technique succeeded, the chest would expand and air would enter the victim's lungs.

The earliest description of mouth-to-mouth resuscitation is in the Bible, when Elisha brought a Shunamite's son back by mouth-to-mouth resuscitation. The story is told in II Kings (4:34):

> And he went up, and lay upon the child, and put his mouth upon his mouth, and his eyes upon his eyes, and his hands upon his hands: and he stretched himself upon the child; and the flesh of the child waxed warm.

The only way to really learn CPR is to take a course of instruction. But here is a general outline.

If you find a collapsed person, first determine if he is conscious by shaking his shoulder and shouting at him. If he does not respond, open his mouth, clearing his airway by pulling on his tongue. The simplest maneuver is the head tilt/neck lift. This is accomplished by putting pressure on the forehead with one hand to extend the head while lifting with the other hand placed under the neck near the back of the head. Just opening the patient's mouth might open the airway and start him breathing. Once the airway is open, place your ear close to the victim's mouth, look at his chest and stomach for movement, and listen for the sounds of breathing. An airway must be supplied; otherwise, oxygen cannot be delivered, and in three to four minutes; time, brain death will occur. (The heart can live without oxygen for twenty minutes, but not the brain.)

Immediately apply your mouth to his mouth for mouth-to-mouth breathing. Pinch the victim's nose shut while keeping the heel of the hand in place to maintain the head in position. Give four quick full breaths in rapid succession. Next, locate the victim's pulse in the neck (the carotid pulse), to see if the heart is beating; slip the tips of your index and middle fingers into the groove between the trachea and the neck muscle, some two inches to the side, to feel the pulse. If no pulse is evident, you must provide artificial circulation in addition to the breathing.

Once it is established that there is no pulse, apply rhythmic pressure on the lower half of the victim's breastbone. Kneel at the victim's side, near his chest, locate the lower portion of the breastbone (sternum), place the heel of one hand about one and a half inches above the tip of the breastbone. Place your other hand on top of this one. Be sure to keep your fingers on the chest wall. Bring your shoulders directly over the victim's breastbone as you press downward. Keep your arms straight. Depress the sternum about one-half inch for an adult. Relaxation must follow the compression immediately and be of equal time. Do not remove your hands from the victim's breastbone while you are allowing the chest to return to its normal position between compressions. If you are the only rescuer, you must provide both the breathing and the cardiac massage. Compress the chest fifteen consecutive times at a rate of 80 beats a minute, followed by two breaths in rapid succession. If there is another rescuer to help you, then one of you should be responsible for breathing, the other for chest compression.

Ventricular fibrillation is a total irregularity, a chaotic action of the heart that occurs at times of cardiac arrest. These lethal arrhythmias have not been successfuly treated with medical therapy, except by the use of defibrillation or cardiac massage.

A brilliant breakthrough took place on February 4, 1980, at the Johns Hopkins Hospital in Baltimore, Maryland, when the first human implantable *cardioverter defibrillator* was inserted. This is an instrument that automatically electrically shocks the heart when it develops a chaotic rhythm. By December, 1983, there were twenty implant centers in the United States and one in Paris, and the total number of individuals who have received this type of implant defibrillator exceeded two hundred and twenty. This remarkable instrument was devised by Dr. Michael Mirowski, who is presently at the department of medicine in Sinai Hospital in Baltimore.

Whenever ventricular fibrillation occurs, this device delivers twenty-five jolts of electricity, some fifteen to twenty seconds after the onset of the irregularity. A special lithium battery provides an estimated monitoring life of three years, or one hundred discharges. The device can be tested by a magnet when attached to a test load resistor, rather than having to open the chest.

The patients who receive the internal defibrillator are those who have had one or more episodes of ventricular fibrillation and are at risk to have further episodes.

ESTABLISHING BREATHLESSNESS

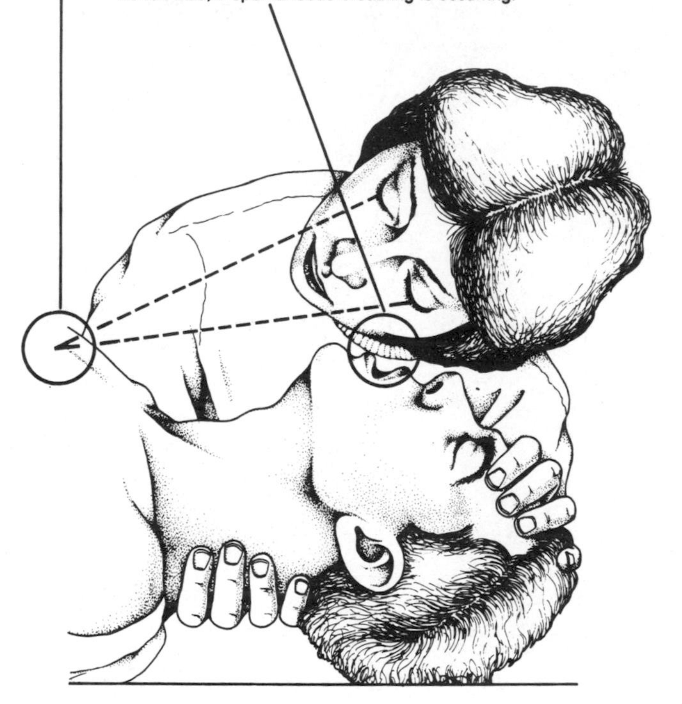

Assess the victim in this manner for 10-15 seconds. If breathing is present, maintain the airway position and check for pulses. If breathing is absent, administer rescue breaths.

RESCUE BREATHING

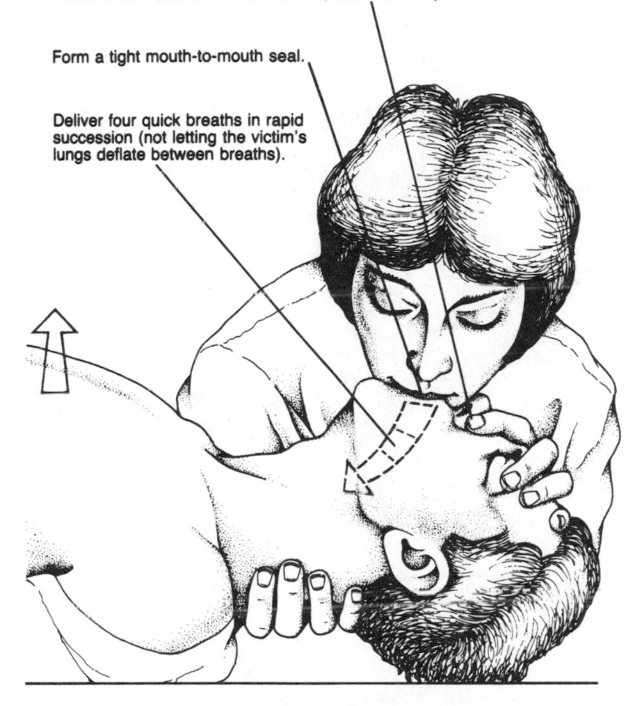

After this blast of four rescue breaths, glance at the chest, which should begin to fall as exhalation occurs—and again, exhaled air may be sensed by the cheek. Then:

- If successful, proceed to check pulses.
- If unsuccessful, reposition the airway and try one more time.
- If effective ventilation is still lacking, assume that the upper airway is obstructed, and proceed to clear it.

CHECKING PULSES

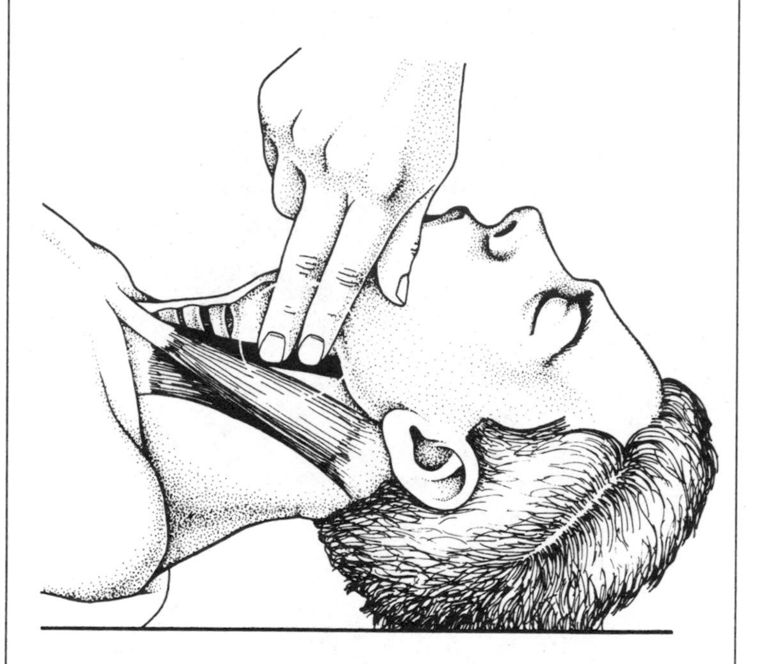

Palpate for the carotid pulse with two fingers between the thyroid cartilage, anterior edge of the sternocleidomastoid muscle, and mandible. *Remember:* Try the opposite side (quickly) if no pulse is appreciated. In hospital patients, the femoral pulse may be checked below the inguinal ligament's middle third.

- If pulses are present, continue rescue breathing until spontaneous ventilation resumes (or until help arrives and the airway can be managed more definitively).
- If pulses are absent, begin full CPR.

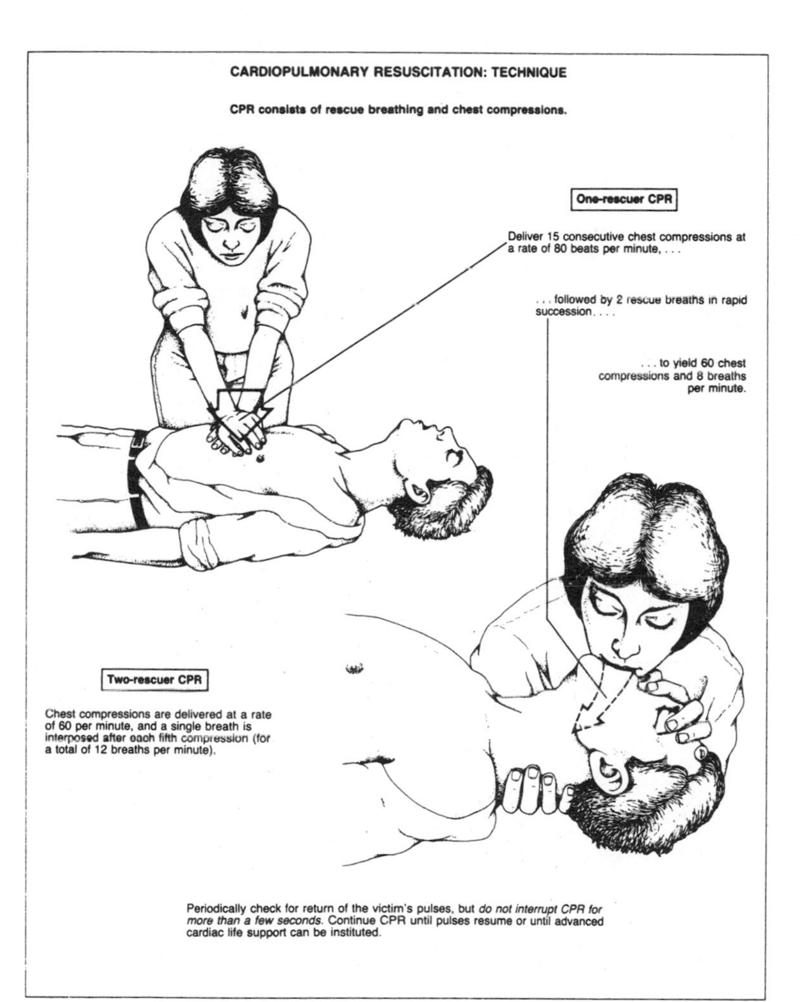
CARDIOPULMONARY RESUSCITATION: TECHNIQUE
CPR consists of rescue breathing and chest compressions.
One-rescuer CPR
Deliver 15 consecutive chest compressions at a rate of 80 beats per minute, . . .
. . . followed by 2 rescue breaths in rapid succession, . . .
. . . to yield 60 chest compressions and 8 breaths per minute.
Two-rescuer CPR
Chest compressions are delivered at a rate of 60 per minute, and a single breath is interposed after each fifth compression (for a total of 12 breaths per minute).
Periodically check for return of the victim's pulses, but do not interrupt CPR for more than a few seconds. Continue CPR until pulses resume or until advanced cardiac life support can be instituted.

Index